Community Health
Promotion Ideas
That Work

The Jones and Bartlett Series in Health

Community Health Promotion Ideas That Work

A Field-Book for Practitioners

Marshall W. Kreuter
Health 2000
Atlanta, Georgia

Nicole A. Lezin
Health 2000
Atlanta, Georgia

Matthew W. Kreuter
St. Louis University
St. Louis, Missouri

Lawrence W. Green
University of British Columbia
Vancouver, BC, Canada

JONES AND BARTLETT PUBLISHERS
Sudbury, Massachusetts
BOSTON   TORONTO   LONDON   SINGAPORE

World Headquarters

Jones and Bartlett Publishers
40 Tall Pine Drive
Sudbury, MA 01776
978-443-5000
info@jbpub.com
www.jbpub.com

Jones and Bartlett Publishers Canada
P.O. Box 19020
Toronto, ON M5S 1X1
CANADA

Jones and Bartlett Publishers International
Barb House, Barb Mews
London W6 7PA
UK

Library of Congress Cataloging-in-Publication Data
Community health promotion ideas that work : a field-book for
    practitioners / Marshall W. Kreuter . . . [et al.].
        p.   cm.
    Includes bibliographical references and index.
    ISBN 0-7637-0408-3
    1. Health promotion. 2. Health promotion—Case studies.
I. Kreuter, Marshall W.
RA427.8.C636 1997
362.l'2—dc21   97-3555
                                                              CIP

Vice President and Acquisitions Editor: Joseph E. Burns
Production Editor: Martha Stearns
Manufacturing Buyer: Jenna Sturgis
Design and Editorial Production Service: WordCrafters Editorial Services, Inc.
Typesetting: WordCrafters Editorial Services, Inc.
Cover Design: Hannus Design Associates
Printing and Binding: Edwards Brothers, Inc.
Cover Printing: John P. Pow Company

Printed in the United States of America
02   01   00   99   98   10   9   8   7   6   5   4   3   2

Contents

Chapter 6   TACTICS   145

Chapter 7   STEERING VS. ROWING   187

List of Figures

List of Tables

Acknowledgments

This book is a tribute to the ideas and successes of many people within the field of public health. The researchers and practitioners who have shared their findings with us, directly or through their published work and teaching, are acknowledged in the text. In addition, there are many others whose actions and ideas have profoundly influenced this book. We realize that any listing will be incomplete; any omissions are unintended and should be attributed to our failing memories!

We express our respectful gratitude to David Altman, Zhang Baoyi, Bill Beery, Teresa Byrd, Ellen Capwell, Steve Coen, Billie Corti, David Cotton, Donna Cross, Delisa Culpepper, Jim Dale, Lori Dorfman, Michael Eriksen, Steve Fawcett, Bill Foege, Stu Fors, Bob Gold, Yu Hai, Jim Herrington, Peter Howatt, Grade Imoh, Steve Jones, Bob Kingon, Adam Koplan, Fred Kroger, Brick Lancaster, Richard Levinson, Dave Lohrmann, Bob Moon, Chuck Nelson, Hod Ogden, Guy Parcel, Kathy Parker, Joe Patterson, Ken Powell, Pekka Puska, Amelie Ramirez, Glen Ray, Gayle Reiber, Barbara Rimer, Mark Rosenberg, Randy Schwartz, Vic Strecker, Marni Vliet, Larry Wallack, Nancy Watkins, Lynna Williams, Susan Zaro, and Dexiu Zhang.

We would like to thank the many friends and colleagues who agreed to be photographed as the composite characters depicted in the case stories: Drew Baughman, Ken Castro, Michele Chang, Charlie Chen, David Cotton, Sara Craig, Teresa Durden, Adele Franks, Mary Jenssen, Bob Kingon, Adam Koplan, Arthur Lezin, Linda Miller, Ron Miller, Bobby Milstein, Bob Pinner, Erika Reed, and Bob Robinson. Their good-natured cooperation with our somewhat unusual request enlivens the text and helps us convey visually the human side of the stories we tried to capture in writing. Troy Hall, who took each of the photographs, somehow found exactly the right expression for each portrait. His technical skills with lights and lenses are paralleled by his ability to make his subjects relax and laugh.

Our publisher, Joe Burns of Jones and Bartlett Publishers, encouraged us throughout the project with his enthusiasm for the book's content and a clear sense of its audience.

Sonja Greene deserves special recognition for her patience and skillful work throughout the long production process. Unfazed by voluminous changes, lost diskettes, hand-scribbled graphics, and elusive citations, she graciously and persistently kept us on track and on schedule. This book would never have moved beyond outlines and enticing first paragraphs without her. She is perhaps more relieved than the authors and publishers that it is finally done!

As always, our time-consuming labors are possible only through the support of those closest to us: Martha, Jack, Tricia, and Judith.

Introduction

In trying to explain what he means by a positive notion of health, Leon Kass invites us to ponder this analogy:

> What is a healthy squirrel? Not a picture of a squirrel, not . . . the sleeping squirrel, not even the aggregate of his normal blood pressure, serum calcium, total body zinc, normal digestion, fertility, and the like. Rather, the healthy squirrel is a bushy-tailed fellow who looks and acts like a squirrel; who leaps through trees with great daring; who gathers, buries, and covers but later uncovers and recovers his acorns; who perches out on a limb, who chatters and plays and courts with mates, and rears his young in large improbable-looking homes at the tops of trees. . . .*

By using this metaphor to interpret *health*, Kass suggests that one practical way for us to understand the meaning of something as complex as health is to describe the notion in its whole context and to imagine how it might manifest itself or what it might look like.

In preparing this book, we took Kass's advice and repeatedly asked ourselves: What does effective health promotion look like? This question prompted two others: (1) What do effective health promotion practitioners do? and (2) What ideas or thought processes seem to guide the decisions they make? Out of this repetitive process emerged a variety of actions and ideas, some of which were persistent. We call the persistent ones "ideas that work."

Great progress has been made in health education and health promotion in recent years. Thanks to the combined good work of dedicated practitioners and researchers the world over, we now have a much more coherent picture of what it takes to put into place health promotion programs that work. In our travels and collective work experiences, we have had the great pleasure of observing and working alongside health educators and public health advocates from Boston, Massachusetts, to Lagos, Nigeria; from Bethel, Alaska, to Vancouver, British Columbia; from Perth, Australia, to

---

* Kass LR. Medical care and the pursuit of health. In: Lindsay, C, ed. *New Directions in Public Health Care.* 3rd ed. San Francisco: Institute for Contemporary Studies; 1980: 16–17.

Tianjin, China. It has been inspiring to see these health workers use their ingenuity to create conditions that will put people in a better position to improve their health and quality of life, often operating with meager resources. In spite of this good work, however, a gap remains: the gap between what we know works and what is actually being applied in the name of health education and health promotion. The idea for this book was generated by the persistence of this gap and the desire to narrow it.

Although there are many possible explanations for why this gap persists, one in particular has inspired this book. In localities throughout the world, the profile of the health promotion practitioner is often that of a person who offers great commitment and enthusiasm, but has limited background preparation and/or experience in the complex tasks he or she is being asked to perform. For those frontline workers, we have tried to create a user-friendly book that will impart knowledge gained by other researchers and practitioners, offer specific suggestions to plan and carry out effective health promotion programs, and, most of all, stimulate both thought and discussion about different approaches.

This book is organized into seven chapters, each of which begins with a case story. Although fictional, the case stories are based upon real experiences and include nuances of the human condition that are so often excluded from more scientifically oriented accounts of public health practice. The case stories are intended to provide a practical frame of reference for the critical issues and principles highlighted in each chapter. Epidemiologists often exhort each other to remember the faces behind public health statistics; the case stories in this book represent our attempt to do the same for health promotion practitioners.

Chapter 1: Finding True North

The case story that launches this chapter is entitled "Why Do We Do What We Do?" This rhetorical question asks practitioners to examine the rationale for determining how they spend their time and resources. The case story chronicles the experiences of a young and enthusiastic health worker who plans and implements a health promotion activity that, on the surface, looks fine. However, the case story analysis raises questions that cause us to re-examine whether the activity she chose was the wisest use of resources.

Chapter 2: From Information to Insight

In this chapter's case story, "Making Tough Choices," health department staff struggle to choose from two competing claims on their attention and resources. Ultimately, they must defend their choice before the state legislators who provide funding for their programs. The case story and analysis explore the sources and uses of public health data to determine priorities.

Chapter 3: Discovering the Causes

"What Causes the Causes?" shows how a determined community coalition tackled underage drinking and drug use in its community. By systematically identifying the factors contributing to this serious and complex problem, the coalition is able to identify which factors are most amenable to change. The case analysis helps readers conduct a similar analysis for other health problems in their own communities.

Chapter 4: Promoting Social Capital

In "The Court of Public Opinion," a frustrated, disheartened health department leader gets a pep talk from a friend in the journalism business. The case story and analysis illustrate the importance of communicating about what we do, eliciting meaningful participation, and generating "social capital"—the interactions among us that lead to mutual gain.

Chapter 5: Theory Applied

Experience has taught us that contemporary health problems are most likely to yield to interventions when multiple methods or tactics are matched to the specific needs and unique characteristics of the population. "The Old Horse" takes us to China and illustrates how such a process was successfully carried out. It illustrates how selected theories, in combination with an understanding of cultural phenomena, were used to create an effective health promotion program. The analysis of the case story is followed by summaries of five key theories that belong in the repertoire of every health promotion worker.

Chapter 6: Tactics

The case story that begins this chapter, "Checkmate," uses the analogy of chess to highlight the combination of strategy and tactics used to vanquish an opponent. In the less competitive but more complicated sphere of health promotion, strategy and tactics are also key considerations. The case analysis reviews health communication, media advocacy, and policy tactics that are valuable tools for health promotion practitioners.

Chapter 7: Steering vs. Rowing

In "Jameson," we return to the setting and characters introduced in the first case story, "Why Do We Do What We Do?" In addition to reexamining program priorities described in the first chapter, this question triggers a health department leader to consider the managerial and organizational tenets that provide a solid foundation for effective health promotion work.

To paraphrase the English statesman Lord Acton, "Ignorance and the love of ease are the natural enemies of progress." Our intention is not to create a "cookbook" that makes health education and health promotion easy. Rather, it is to bring into sharper focus the central tasks of health promotion without losing sight of the reason for doing them: health improvement. If readers make those connections, and do so with some ease, so much the better.

Time will judge whether this vision or dream is more or less realized. To the extent that more is achieved, credit will inevitably go to practitioners in the field, for it is our experience that once they are given even a modest amount of support, they rarely settle for less!

Good luck and good health!

> Marshall Kreuter
> Nicole Lezin
> Matthew Kreuter
> Lawrence Green

CHAPTER 1

Finding True North

Case Story
_____ WHY DO WE DO WHAT WE DO? _____

Linda Thomas had prepared for her first-ever presentation at the annual Georgia Public Health Association (GPHA) meeting just like every other task she undertook—with careful attention to details and great enthusiasm. That's the way the Thomas family did things.

In her presentation, Linda described how she had recruited a total of 51 volunteers for a stress reduction program from Clarkston High School and two businesses: the Oconee Garment Manufacturing Company—where most of the volunteers were women who did shift work on sewing machines—and Southern Electronics, a company that manufactures computer components. During the course of a two-month period, she had provided the volunteer participants with six one-hour sessions that included instruction in relaxation techniques, small-group discussions to examine the sources of stress, and instruction in low-impact physical activity.

The results from Linda's evaluation showed that after their participation in the stress management course, participants were much more likely than control-group subjects to identify and manage stressful circumstances. Those who had participated in the course also reported higher job satisfaction than control subjects.

Linda was also elated when a friend invited her to leaf through the comments that some of the participants had written on the session evaluation: "Crisp and to the point." "Handled questions like a pro!" "Great enthusiasm."

At the barbecue social the evening after her presentation, Linda was introduced to Dr. Fran Martin, who was giving the keynote address the following day. Dr. Martin was one of those living legends of public health. Everyone knew who she was: former dean of the University of California School of Public Health at Berkeley and former senior White House advisor. Dr. Martin was most recognized for her courageous work in establishing primary health centers in Mississippi during the 1950s and 1960s. She was now in what she called "semi-retirement." In reality, she was as busy as ever: writing, consulting, and giving presentations such as the one she was delivering the next day.

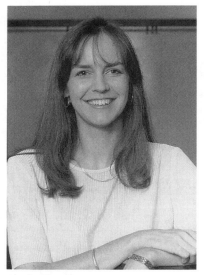

Linda Thomas

"It's really an honor to meet you, Dr. Martin." Linda's sincerity was genuine.

"Just Fran, everyone calls me Fran." She had smiling eyes and an easy manner. "Incidentally, I attended your session today. Enthusiasm like yours is certainly contagious. Hang on to it!" Fran Martin was an engaging person who never seemed to be in a hurry; it was a pleasure to be in her company.

"Thank you. I noticed you in the back of the room toward the end of my presentation. I'm glad I didn't see you earlier, because I would have been even more nervous than I was."

Fran gestured toward a table. "Join me for dinner?"

Linda and Dr. Martin joined three others at a round table with a red-and-white checked paper tablecloth. The dinner conversation was lively and covered everything from gun control to the succulent barbecue. When someone jokingly asked Dr. Martin if she knew the health effects of eating barbecue, she paused, dramatically picked up a small juicy piece of barbecue with her fingers, and declared: "My motto is: All things in moderation, but a taste of something a little *sinful* every now and then!" She promptly popped the morsel into her mouth to a chorus of cheers from her tablemates.

During the dinner conversation, Fran learned that Linda was formerly an elementary-school teacher and had been working as a health educator for the Tri-County Health Department (TCHD) for just under two years. "How did you get interested in stress management?" Fran asked.

"About six months after I joined the Tri-County Health Department, I attended a wellness conference in Florida. I learned that high levels of stress are significant contributors to a variety of health problems and that relatively simple, low-cost exercises can alleviate stress."

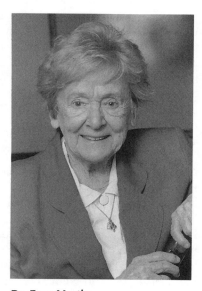

Dr. Fran Martin

Fran gave an understanding nod and Linda continued. "While I was participating in the workshop, I felt the immediate benefits of relaxation and the breathing exercises." And then she lowered her voice to say, "Frankly, what the instructor was doing didn't seem all that complicated."

Fran chuckled. How refreshing it was to observe self-confidence!

Linda went on. "Anyway, after I got back from the wellness conference, I prepared a trip report and included a proposal to do a stress reduction demonstration program for personnel in selected schools and businesses within the Tri-County area."

"And your supervisor thought it was a good idea?" Fran probed.

"Actually, my regular health education supervisor had resigned to take another position and the county was in a hiring freeze, so my county health officer, Dr. Jameson, read the report. He told me that I could undertake the project as long as the program costs didn't have to come from the TCHD budget and if I did it without compromising my workload. Incidentally, Dr. Jameson will be here tomorrow to hear your presentation."

Fran could picture the position Linda's health officer had been in. In Linda, he had an employee with modest public health experience but great potential—a person with high energy and that intuitive knack for seeing and acting on opportunities to make things work. Fran could just imagine that Dr. Jameson wanted to nurture that potential and give her encouragement. Good personnel are hard to find, let alone keep!

The next day, Linda secured a seat in the front row at Dr. Martin's keynote address. The conference host took the podium and, after declaring that Dr. Martin needed no introduction, launched into a lengthy reading of her résumé. During the introduction, Fran caught Linda's eye and winked.

The person introducing Fran finally wound down, ". . .the title of her presentation is: "Priorities for Whom?" Will you please welcome Dr. Fran Martin."

Enthusiastic applause welcomed Dr. Martin. The applause stopped and the room was silent. Fran stood at the podium, looked down at her notes, and then slowly scanned the audience. In a clear, soft voice she asked: "Why do we do what we do?" The room remained silent. Then she asked rhetorically: "By what criteria are the human and economic resources of your organization or group assigned to actions designed to improve the public's health?" Everyone remained silent, awaiting the correct answer. Looking at the audience, she hunched her shoulders and partially extended her arms and asked: "Well?"

After another pause, she continued. "It's an interesting question, don't you think? What would serve as the basis for your response? Would it reflect some systematic assessment of the health needs of those you serve? Would it show that what you are doing is connected to what your organization stands for and is committed to? Would it reveal that the limited time and resources you have at hand are indeed being directed at those things that citizens perceive to be most important to their health?"

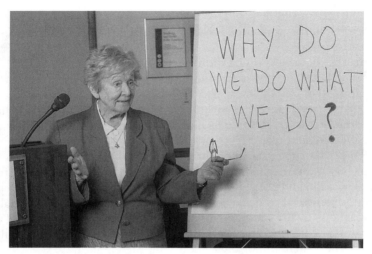

Dr. Fran Martin giving her lecture

Dr. Martin continued. "I find it useful to ask myself regularly: Why do I do what I do? If you remember nothing else in what I have to say this morning, please remember that simple question because I suspect that, like me, you will discover that your responses will lead you to insights you may not otherwise have considered."

The audience listened and thought. It was as if Dr. Martin were talking directly to each one of them. After jotting *Why do we do what we do?* in her notebook, Linda wondered to herself, *Why did I undertake the stress management project?* And she answered herself, *I was informed that stress was an important issue. . . . I found it to be an interesting approach, and those who experienced the program enjoyed it. And I have the interest and the ability to do it!*

Dr. Martin was now into her presentation full swing. She showed slides of data comparing the leading causes of death, disease, and disability in Georgia with those of the rest of the nation. Then she showed a map of the southeastern portion of the United States and indicated that portions of South Carolina and Georgia are in what is called America's "stroke belt." She also pointed out that some of the states' highest rates of infant mortality and teen pregnancy are found in this same area.

She paused and said: "You know, we have very good evidence that carefully planned health promotion programs can do a good deal to prevent these health problems and improve the quality of life not only of those who might otherwise have been needlessly victimized, but of their families as well." Knowing that she wasn't likely to get a response, Dr. Martin added, "Did you all know that?"

Linda fixed her gaze on the map—the Tri-County area was in the stroke belt.

Pointing to the map, Dr. Martin continued. "At the risk of stating the obvious, I think we can do a much better job of putting into place programs that we know work. But to do that, we need to have better information, we need to digest and employ that information, and we need to be more focused." Dr. Martin paused to take a sip of water and then added, "I can't remember who said it. Perhaps I did, long ago. Anyway, this quote seems quite appropriate here: 'The greatest obstacle to discovery is not ignorance, it's the assumption of knowledge.' I want to ask you to think seriously about what this means to your daily work."

As Dr. Martin made her closing remarks, Linda's thoughts darted back and forth between her stress management project and images of people suffering needless death and disability due to stroke and infant mortality. *But my project was so well received,* she thought.

Case Analysis

Most of us can identify with those who try to assemble a complicated device without reading the instructions. We can get just so far before getting stuck, and spend a lot of our time and energy trying to get unstuck! The basic principles of public health offer us important guidance that can minimize the chances of getting stuck and ending up where we don't want to be.

Linda Thomas's experience in "Why Do We Do What We Do?" gives us a context to examine the practical relevance of some of the fundamental principles in public health—principles that are somewhat analogous to the instructions that came with that complicated device.

WHY DID LINDA UNDERTAKE THE STRESS MANAGEMENT PROJECT?

Linda's trip to the wellness conference in Florida was a positive personal experience. She learned that there is evidence linking stress to a variety of health problems. Full of goodwill and good intentions, and armed with an interesting idea, she sought out an opportunity to apply and test her idea. The question she wanted to answer was: If people are taught stress management skills, will they report that the experience was beneficial and worth their while? Based on what we know from the story, the answer to her question was generally positive. Linda's experience is a good example of social learning theory in action. She had learned a new skill, gained confidence that she could use it, and demonstrated that she could apply it. Positive personal experiences are strong motivators; indeed, we tend to act on those things we do well, especially when our efforts are received with praise.

The story forces us to acknowledge that while Linda was carrying out her stress management effort, another public health problem was apparently not being addressed. We know that the area served by the Tri-County Health Department had high rates of stroke, hypertension, infant mortality, and teen pregnancy. We heard Dr. Martin mention that the public health literature indicates that health promotion and disease prevention approaches have been effective in addressing the problems of stroke, hypertension, infant mortality, and teen pregnancy. Here's the picture: We have a population where we can document priority health problems that affect a large number of people, and we have knowledge of effective interventions for these problems—but we have taken no apparent action. This raises a legitimate question: In the face of this information, was Linda's work on the stress management project the most appropriate use of her time and energy as a Tri-County Health Department health educator?

WHAT DO DR. JAMESON'S ACTIONS TELL US?

Linda Thomas is obviously a talented, energetic woman—all the more reason that her talents and energies should be focused on those activities most likely to have the greatest health benefit for the community served by the health department. But apparently no one, including her health officer, Dr. Jameson, raised the issue of the public health importance of what Linda was proposing to do. Why not?

Fran Martin had correctly assessed the position Dr. Jameson had been in: he knew that Linda was a potentially outstanding employee and apparently didn't want to discourage the initiative and enthusiasm she had demonstrated. What we don't know from the story is whether the Tri-County Health Department had a conceptual plan in place that would (1) help everyone see the direction in which the department was headed, and (2) guide the distribution of its limited resources to the priority health problems and priority prevention strategies within its service area.

Box 1.1, "Public Health in America," provides us with a general example of the key components of such a plan. It shows (1) the vision and mission of public health, (2) the six primary functions of public health, and (3) ten public health services deemed to be essential. The vision of healthy people in healthy communities reflects the condition that public health scientists and practitioners hope to achieve. The mission tells us how the vision will be achieved—through health promotion and disease, injury, and disability prevention. The six functions and the ten essential services indicate the actions or tasks that need to be carried out by public health workers. Note that the first two essential services listed involve assessing a community's health needs and investigating the determinants of health problems.

The public health perspective shown in Box 1.1 reveals a fundamental public health assumption: assessment of local needs is essential because health problems and their causes vary from community to community. For

Box 1.1
PUBLIC HEALTH IN AMERICA

Vision

Healthy people in healthy communities

Mission

Promote physical and mental health and
prevent disease, injury, and disability

Public Health Functions

- Prevent epidemics and the spread of disease
- Protect against environmental hazards
- Prevent injuries
- Promote and encourage healthy behaviors and mental health
- Respond to disasters and assist communities in recovery
- Assure the quality and accessibility of health services

Essential Public Health Services

- Monitor health status to identify and solve community health problems
- Diagnose and investigate health problems and health hazards in the community
- Inform, educate, and empower people about health issues
- Mobilize community partnerships and action to solve health problems
- Develop policies and plans that support individual and community health efforts
- Enforce laws and regulations that protect health and ensure safety
- Link people to needed personal health services and assure the provision of health care when otherwise unavailable
- Assure a competent workforce
- Evaluate effectiveness, accessibility, and quality of personal and population-based health services
- Research new insights and innovative solutions to health problems

Source: Baker EL, Melton RJ, Strange PV, et al. Health reform and the health of the public: forging community health partnerships. *JAMA.* 1994;272:1276–1282.

example, the most prevalent health problems of children in rural Nigeria (malaria, diarrhea, lack of immunization) are not likely to be the same as those observed among children in Atlanta, Georgia (injuries, violence).

If the Tri-County Health Department did not have such a plan, it should have. If it did have a plan, it was Dr. Jameson's responsibility to make sure that all members of the TCHD, including Linda, understood what their organization's priorities were and why they were important.

Who wouldn't appreciate Dr. Jameson's support of Linda's display of initiative, considering the resignation of the area health education supervisor and the constraints on the Tri-County Health Department's budget? However, Dr. Jameson did Linda no favor by letting her move forward with so little counsel. One of the primary tasks of a supervisor is to help employees channel their good ideas and enthusiasm into directions that will help fulfill the vision and mission of the organization. Clearly, Dr. Jameson's decision to let Linda move forward with her idea without a critical review of the options is an important part of this story, but it is not the whole story. There is a lesson here for everyone, practitioners *and* managers. In the delivery of public health services, the reality is that we cannot do it all. With limited time and resources, the provision of services must be driven by rational criteria. Such criteria are reflected in such simple questions as:

What are the documented needs of the people we serve?

What are the perceived needs of the people we serve?

What works?

How does this proposed initiative fit in with the mission of our agency?

What economic and human resources are available?

Most health promotion practitioners work in and for organizations like public health departments, volunteer agencies, schools, or businesses. All of these entities have explicit purposes and goals, which are usually reflected in their organizational mission statements. An organization's mission statement describes what the organization is trying to accomplish and how it intends to go about it. Look again at the mission statement for public health cited in Box 1.1.

Typically, a mission statement builds on previous attempts to define the scope and purpose of public health activities. Why is this important if each public health agency must address unique community needs? A common mission is important precisely because the number of problems an organization could potentially address far exceeds its capacity to address them all. Thus, if health workers understand and share a common vision and mission of their organization, they are more likely to be focused on priority issues and to be in sync with one another.

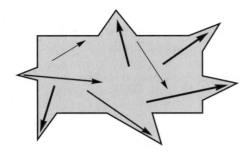

FIGURE 1.1   Unaligned Team

Boston Celtics basketball hall-of-famer Bill Russell has some sage advice to offer. He said that although the Celtics were a group of highly skilled specialists, their success depended ". . .both on individual excellence and how well we worked together."[1] Two figures graphically illustrate different scenarios.[2] In Figure 1.1, the arrows going in different directions reflect a group or team in which the members are out of alignment. Even though the individuals may work hard and have the best of intentions, their collective effort as a team would likely be incoherent and inefficient.

In Figure 1.2, the alignment of the arrows suggests the kind of coherence and common purpose one would expect among members of an organization that share a common vision and mission.

Even when our role in an organization may be narrowly defined (*e.g.*, adult health and chronic disease, school health, inspecting restaurants, immunizing children), vision and mission statements give us a framework for explaining how the specific tasks we perform fit into a larger picture—in other words, why we do what we do.

In 1988, the authors of *The Future of Public Health* described three core functions of public health: assessment, policy development, and assurance.[3] These functions, which are incorporated into the essential services listed in Box 1.1, are defined as follows:[4]

Assessment:

The regular collection, analysis and sharing of information about health conditions, risks and resources in a community. The

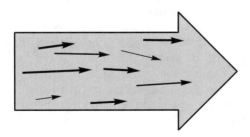

FIGURE 1.2   Aligned Team

assessment function is needed to identify trends in illness, injury and death, the factors which may cause these events, available health resources and their application, unmet needs and community perceptions about health issues.
Short definition: Figuring out what the important health problems are.

Policy Development:

The process whereby public health agencies evaluate and determine health needs and the best ways to address them.
Short definition: Deciding what to do.

Assurance:

Making sure that the needed health services and functions are available.
Short definition: Making it available and doing it right.

The core functions of public health reveal public health's broader framework and distinguish what is unique and invaluable about what public health workers do. To see how these ideas are translated into reality, let's consider a well-documented detective story.[5] On January 12, 1993, officials of a Seattle hospital notified the Washington State Public Health Department that they had recorded increased visits for bloody diarrhea and that three children had been hospitalized with hemolytic uremic syndrome (HUS) and had confirmed a strain of bacteria known as *Escherichia coli* 0157:H7, hereafter referred to as *E. coli*. This strain of *E. coli* produces a powerful toxin that causes severe illness manifested by painful abdominal cramps and diarrhea, which is sometimes bloody. In most cases, *E. coli* infection results from consuming undercooked ground beef. The bacteria are present in the stool of infected persons and can be spread if proper hygienic practices are not followed. Among children and the elderly, it can lead to the destruction of red blood cells, acute kidney failure, seizures, stroke, and even death.

On January 15, the health department initiated active surveillance throughout the greater Seattle area. By January 17, interviews with 37 patients revealed that 27 of them had eaten hamburgers from a particular fast-food chain. The interviews revealed that the hamburgers had been consumed in different outlets of the same fast-food chain. On January 18, Washington State public health officials made a public announcement of the findings from a case-control study confirming that the cause of the outbreak was the result of the food preparation methods of a specific fast-food chain, wherein the meat processing had been improper and the hamburger patties had been undercooked. The announcement was accompanied with health

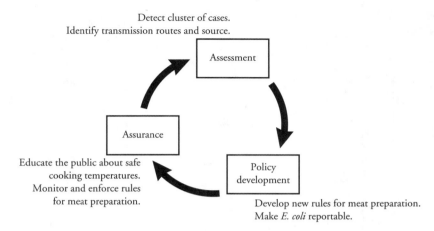

FIGURE 1.3   The Core Functions Applied

education messages alerting food service workers and the general public about the need to cook hamburger meat thoroughly.

Immediately after the January 18 announcement, the fast-food chain voluntarily removed the hamburger from its restaurants. In total, the outbreak resulted in 501 people becoming ill, three of whom died. Epidemiologists estimated that the action to remove 250,000 potentially contaminated hamburgers prevented at least 800 additional cases of illness. Thus, 800 persons who would most certainly have gotten sick, some of whom may have died, didn't. Interestingly, we cannot know who those 800 people were. This provides a good example of why public health is often referred to as "the silent miracle." In a society where sensational media coverage predominates our intellectual landscape, most of the media attention to the Seattle outbreak focused on the fast food, not the timely and effective response of public health workers.

As Figure 1.3 shows, the core functions of public health in Washington State worked! Through a vigilant and active assessment, they detected a serious problem and tracked down its cause. Policy development enabled *E. coli* to be reportable and created systems to assure approved meat sources, proper cooking procedures, and timely public education.

Figure 1.4 shows the dramatic rise and fall of the *E. coli* outbreak. Behind these numbers and bars are real people, real families, and a real community. While there may be some who cynically view the three core functions of assurance, assessment, and policy development as esoteric descriptors, we suspect that the people of Seattle see it differently. It is understanding this broader picture of community health work that will help Linda Thomas keep her efforts focused in the future.

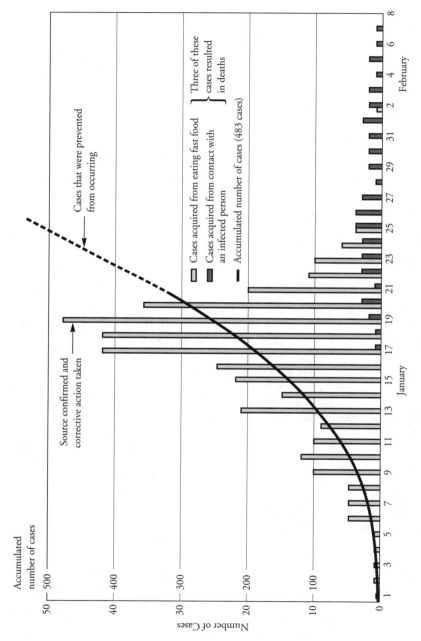

FIGURE 1.4 The Rise and Fall of *E. coli* Cases

HOW WOULD YOU ASSESS THE APPROACH LINDA TOOK IN IMPLEMENTING HER STRESS MANAGEMENT PROJECT?

As you consider this question, keep in mind the second and fourth points under "Public Health Functions" in Box 1.1: *Protect against environmental hazards* and *Promote and encourage healthy behaviors and mental health.* Again, Linda deserves high marks for her enthusiasm and her ability to work with multiple organizations to plan, implement, and evaluate a program. Based on the limited information in the case story, it appears that Linda's approach was exclusively focused on promoting healthful behavior among the volunteers—equipping them with knowledge and skills enabling them to manage stress. However, we see no evidence that she took into account the conditions and environmental circumstances that might be giving rise to the stress the volunteers were trying to control. Is it possible that working conditions in the garment factory (*e.g.,* temperature, noise, time on the shift, potential risk of injury) may have contributed to volunteer stress?

Had Linda considered the extent to which working conditions contribute to stress in the workplace, her approach would likely have been different. Behavioral science and educational theory, confirmed by empirical studies, suggests that the immediate effect of her approach and the sustainability of that effect, would have been improved had Linda examined possible sources of stress in the environment and then moved to ameliorate them.

Unless an organization makes the commitment to institutionalize an educational program as a standard benefit, it will, like so many other efforts, be a one-time-only demonstration. Had the removal of environmental stressors been part of the approach Linda took, benefits gained through environmental changes could be sustained over time; those same benefits would also be enjoyed by newer employees who had not experienced the stress management program.

This is not at all to say that Linda's individual-skills approach was without merit—clearly, employees will benefit from new insights and competencies that they can use outside as well as inside the workplace. What did Linda use as a frame of reference for planning her stress management effort?

We have found it useful to encourage practitioners to examine the basic assumptions they make when developing an intervention plan. Organizational management specialists sometimes refer to these basic assumptions as *mental models*[6] and describe them as pictures we carry in our minds. These subconscious pictures influence how we see the world and, consequently, the actions we take.

We can only surmise what Linda Thomas's mental model was when she first began to imagine the possibility of creating a stress management program. Our attempt to paint a picture of a mental model that reflects a public health perspective follows.

Picture 1

It is true that certain behaviors (*e.g.*, smoking, consumption of high-fat foods, drinking alcohol and driving, not following a prescribed medical regimen, etc.) increase the risks for ill health and that changing these behaviors can reduce the risks.

Picture 2

It is also true that environmental forces, including the living conditions in and out of the workplace, play a substantial role in influencing those behaviors.

Picture 3

Thus, any health promotion approach that fails to take into account the extent to which social and environmental factors may influence individual and collective behavior is likely to have a limited effect.

REALISTICALLY, CAN A STAFF PERSON HAVE ANY INFLUENCE ON SETTING PROGRAM PRIORITIES?

Like many public health promotion practitioners, Linda Thomas works in a bureaucratic organization where the primary means of obtaining collective input is through department or unit staff meetings. During these meetings, even the most junior staff person has the opportunity for input through several means: (1) submitting or recommending an agenda item, (2) submitting written comments on a position paper or proposal, and (3) engaging in discussion during the meeting, including asking for points of clarification on matters of priority setting. Those who act on these opportunities share two characteristics. The first is a mental model of public health practice that is in sync with the public health perspective revealed in Box 1.1. The second is simple: a willingness to raise questions and learn. Although the latter characteristic came naturally for Linda, she apparently came up short on the former. Practitioners who view themselves as participants and are aware of and respect the principles of public health will have no problem.

SUMMARY

Dr. Martin's opening rhetorical question is meant to give us all a nudge; it challenges us to articulate the assumptions behind our decisions and to make sure that they are sound and defensible. It is a question that all practitioners, not just newcomers like Linda Thomas, need to call to mind more often. Our failure to ask, "Why do I do what I do?" is not surprising when you think about it. The demands of our daily work routine tend to push our ultimate goals and purposes into the background. It is in such circumstances that we find ourselves driven by the question of, "How should we do this?" rather than, "Why is this important?

This process of inquiry is a continuous one; we don't suddenly arrive at an answer that maps out our daily activities for the next five years. Assumptions and the decisions that flow from them can and should be adapted to changing conditions.

What does this have to do with identifying sources of information and obtaining data? *Assumptions should be based on the best available data.* As public health practitioners, we have a responsibility to be familiar with the broad picture of health status in our communities—a picture, as we know, that Linda Thomas had not yet painted for herself. (If she had, she would have known of and thought about the stroke belt and its implications for her proposed use of resources.) We also have an obligation to obtain relevant data if they are not immediately available, and to apply them skillfully to the problem we are trying to solve.

Finally, a wide gulf often exists between perceived and real threats to community health. Would you guess that more women die each year from breast cancer or lung cancer? Many people would guess that more lives are lost to breast cancer, but they would be wrong. A person who has lost a family member to breast cancer is naturally convinced that breast cancer prevention and treatment efforts should be a priority; however, the family affected by diabetes may feel equally strong about resources for the disease that has ravaged them. Is one more important than the other? Not necessarily. But we often have to choose among equally compelling needs. Data on the relative impact of risk factors and diseases can be one tool in justifying the use of public resources to address community health problems. Only with a solid data-driven foundation can we then contribute meaningfully to broader efforts: setting priorities, allocating scarce resources, and, last but certainly not least, knowing whether our efforts are improving the health status of people in our communities. These issues are addressed in the next chapter.

ENDNOTES

1. Russell W, Branch T. *Second Wind: Memoirs of an Opinionated Man.* New York: Random House; 1979.
2. These diagrams were taken from: Senge P. *The Fifth Discipline.* New York: Doubleday; 1990: 234–235.
3. *The Future of Public Health.* Washington, DC: National Academy Press; 1988.
4. These definitions of the "core functions" have been taken from: *Public Health Improvement Plan: A Progress Report,* Washington State Department of Health, March 1994. We found this document to be an excellent and practical blueprint for strengthening the capacity for public health. For a copy, contact: Office of the Secretary, 1112 SE Quince Street, P.O. Box 47890, Olympia, Washington 98504-7890.

5. Technical information on this example of an *E. coli* infection outbreak was taken from a paper written by Dr. Beth Bell and her colleagues: Bell B, Goldoft M, Griffin P, et al. A multistate outbreak of *E. coli* 0157:H7-associated bloody diarrhea and hemolytic uremic syndrome from hamburgers. *JAMA*. 1994; 272: 1349–1353.

6. Again, we refer you to Peter Senge's *The Fifth Discipline*. In Chapter 10 he provides a detailed description of mental models. Time spent thinking about your mental model for health promotion planning, implementation, and evaluation would be well spent.

CHAPTER 2

From Information to Insight

Case Story
MAKING TOUGH CHOICES

Prologue

Governmental health agencies at the national, regional (state and provincial), and local levels have much in common. Although their organizational configurations and economic bases may vary, all share a common goal: health promotion and disease prevention. They also share a common problem: finite resources available to address health problems that often seem infinite. This reality requires public health agencies to establish priorities to guide their allocation of limited resources. The gulf that so often exists between the magnitude of health problems and an agency's capacity to respond to those problems provides the context for the case story that follows.

Before reviewing the case story, however, readers may find it helpful to review how government checks and balances influence the allocation of public health resources.[1] Each year, state governments are required to pass into law a state budget. Usually there are two elements to a budget: (1) the costs for maintaining existing programs and services, and (2) the proposed costs for new initiatives. In this process, the executive branch of government (the governor) generates a budget based on needs reported by the directors of state government departments (*e.g.,* education, transportation, health and human services, etc.). The governor's budget is then sent as a proposed bill to a body of the state legislature, usually a budget appropriations committee. Based on budget hearings and other discussions and debate, the committee modifies the budget and proposes legislative approval of the amended bill. More debate and compromise follow, until the bill finally passes through the legislative process and is returned to the governor to sign into law.

A key stage in this process occurs just prior to the governor's preparation of the initial budget bill. As mentioned, all state agency directors are asked to document the budgetary needs of their agencies. Like other agen-

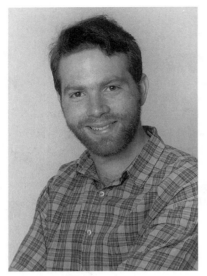

Archie Graham

cies, the health department's success in securing its budget depends on the strength of its proposal. Even though the budget process is political, the importance of providing credible evidence to support program priorities cannot be overemphasized. For public health agencies, this should include epidemiology-based documentation of population risk and evidence that the proposed program, if supported, can work.

Staff Meeting

Archie Graham grabbed a bagel from the passing tray and listened as Jeanine Turner, the department secretary, reviewed the minutes from last month's staff meeting. Staff meetings of the state health department's Health Promotion branch in no way resembled the stereotypical picture of a gathering of bureaucrats. They were focused, lively, informative encounters that relied on staff input and participation.

Elaine Elkins had reported on the success and statewide media coverage of a series of sting operations identifying businesses selling tobacco products to underage youth. Bruce Willett from Biostatistics had presented the sampling plan for the behavioral risk factor survey to be conducted in April. Margie O'Bannon had provided an update on House Bill 462, State Senator Wilma Reeve's proposed measure to create a statewide osteoporosis prevention program to be housed in the Division of Rheumatic Diseases. And finally, to great laughter from everyone around the table, Jeanine reminded the staff that last month's meeting had ended with Bill Minor gloating about his upcoming ski trip to Colorado. Bill, back from his trip and still wearing a cast to his knee, laughed harder than anyone.

It was a good group to work with, and even though Archie had been on board for only six months, he felt like part of the team. Much of the credit for that belonged to the person who had assembled this group, Judith Westphal. Dr. Westphal was branch chief for the Health Promotion/ Chronic Disease Prevention (HPCDP) branch of the state health department. She was an experienced public health worker who had originally been trained as a public health nurse and later had completed graduate degrees in public health education and epidemiology. She was recognized by her supervisor, Dr. Joseph Jackson, and by the workers in her branch as a consummate supervisor. She had high expectations of her staff, but always provided them with whatever support and guidance were necessary to ensure that their tasks could be successfully completed. She involved the staff in decision making. She delegated important projects to them and gave them responsibility and autonomy to complete the work. When giving assignments, she provided clear instructions and set reasonable deadlines.

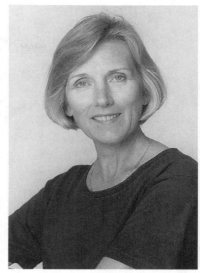

Judith Westphal had led the HPCDP branch since its inception three years ago, when it was established as a new organizational component in the state health department during a reorganization. HPCDP was formed by combining the health education unit, which was part of the director's office, with three other programs: smoking and tobacco, cardiovascular health, and cancer control. At

Dr. Judith Westphal

today's branch meeting, Dr. Westphal would be discussing the HPCDP budget proposal for the next fiscal year. She thanked Jeanine Turner for reviewing the minutes from last month's meeting, welcomed everyone back from the holiday, and offered up extra copies of the meeting agenda for any members who had forgotten theirs.

"As you all know," she began, "it's time to start thinking about next year's budget. The good news is, it looks like the state is going to give us enough funding to continue all the programs and services we already have in place, including the new Lean Choices project. The bad news is, the pool of resources for new initiatives will be much smaller than it has been in past years. Chances are, there'll be only enough money for one or two new projects in the whole department of health."

She continued. "We've had good luck competing for these funds in the past, with Lean Choices last year, and Healthy Seniors two years ago. I talked with Dr. Jackson yesterday to see if he had a particular project in mind for the new initiative funding or if he'd heard of any special topics the state legislators might be favorable toward, and he said he hadn't. He assured me that all reasonable proposals from the branches would be considered for inclusion in the department's final budget. So, even though the odds may be against it, I want us to pursue another new initiative project this year. I've done some preliminary thinking about this, and I'd like us to explore two specific options: breast cancer screening for lower-income women, and some kind of health education program to prevent smokeless tobacco use among youth."

She looked at Archie. "Archie, I'd like you to help me assemble and review the data on both problems, to help determine which one ought to be our top priority. We can discuss our findings at next month's staff meeting,

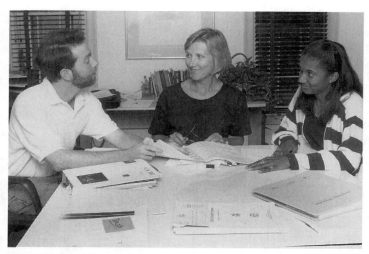

The HPCDP staff meeting

make a decision, and still have plenty of time to put together a solid proposal."

After the meeting, Judith Westphal called Archie into her office and
confided that the task she had given him was of utmost importance. She
explained that virtually all the new initiatives that had been funded in the
past five years were those in which the importance of the problem was
unequivocal and the proposed intervention was shaped by a thorough
understanding of the risk factors and populations at risk. She asked Archie
to take lead responsibility for reviewing the available epidemiologic data on
the two problems. She told him, "If Dr. Jackson sees this proposal as a priority for the department—and I fully expect that he will—I want to make
sure he has more than just our good intentions to back him up when he is
questioned by the governor's office and the appropriations committee . . . you
follow?"

"Got it," Archie replied. He liked working for Judith Westphal—
respect begets respect.

Initial Review of the Data

Two days later, Judith and Archie met again. Although the task for Archie
was fairly well defined—to assess the relative importance of the two health
problems being considered for the new HPCDP initiative—there were many
data sources to consider. Judith suggested that Archie look not only for morbidity and mortality data, but also risk factor data, trend analyses, and data
comparing the extent of each problem in the state to the extent of the problem in neighboring states and elsewhere in the United States. Further, she

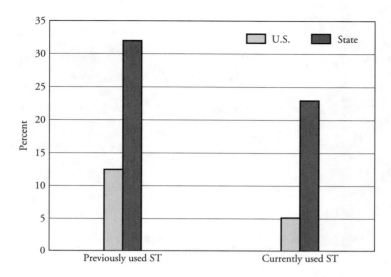

FIGURE 2.1 U.S. and State Prevalence of Previous and Current Use of Smokeless Tobacco (ST) Among Males Age 17 and Older, 1987

advised Archie to seek out local (state) data where it was available, and data that could be stratified by important subgroups within the populations affected. Archie already knew how to access some health data from his days of conducting biannual needs assessments for county health departments, and Judith's suggestions and contacts gave him other ideas, too.

So Archie set out to review as much data as he could find on breast cancer screening, smokeless tobacco use, and the state population. Phone calls to the health statistics branch of the health department and to a local chapter of the American Cancer Society proved especially helpful; within a few days, Archie began receiving some of the information he had requested.

Looking at the data he received on smokeless tobacco use, Archie was surprised at how much higher the rates were in his state compared to others. As a health educator who'd worked in the field for five years, he was well aware that many teenage boys and young men used chewing tobacco and snuff, but he'd never realized how different his state was from others in this respect. In the United States, 12.6 percent of males age seventeen and over had ever used smokeless tobacco, compared to 31.9 percent in his state. While only 5.2 percent of U.S. males were present smokeless tobacco users, nearly one in four (23.1 percent) males in his state were present users (see Figure 2.1).

Archie knew that most adult cigarette smokers begin smoking when they are teenagers, and figured the same might be true of smokeless tobacco users. He was right. In his state, over half (51.3 percent) of smokeless tobacco users had started using smokeless tobacco before age 16, and more than

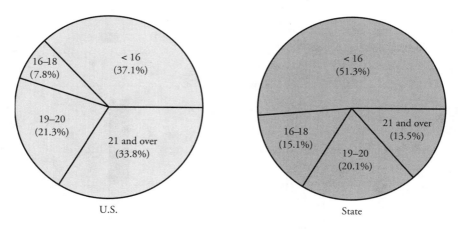

FIGURE 2.2   U.S. and State Age at Initiation
of Smokeless Tobacco Use, 1989

85 percent started before age 21 (see Figure 2.2). As he digested this chart, Archie couldn't help thinking about prevention programs he could propose to Judith to help keep kids from starting to use smokeless tobacco. But he caught himself, knowing that there was much more data to consider and that thinking about interventions at this point was premature.

Archie looked over the data tables that described the demographic characteristics of smokeless tobacco users in the United States (see Tables 2.1 through 2.6). He saw that most smokeless tobacco users were White, young, had a high-school education or less, and tended to be poor. He wished he had similar data for his state, though he doubted there would be any major differences.

For mammography and breast cancer, Archie found that breast cancer rates for Blacks[2] and Whites were roughly the same for women under age 50, but higher for Whites among those age 50 and older (see Figure 2.3). For both age groups, the rates in his state were similar to rates in the United States. But while White women seemed more likely to get breast cancer, Black women were more likely to die from it. For women under age 60, Blacks had higher mortality rates than Whites in all age categories (see Figure 2.4).

TABLE 2.1   U.S. Demographic Characteristics of Smokeless Tobacco (ST) Users,
by Race, 1988

Race	% Previous ST Users	% Current ST Users
White	11.1	5.6
Black	6.6	3.0
Other	7.7	2.9

TABLE 2.2   U.S. Demographic Characteristics of Smokeless Tobacco (ST) Users, by Age, 1988

Age	% Previous ST Users	% Current ST Users
17–19	12.3	8.2
20–29	11.4	5.9
30–39	7.3	4.1
40–49	9.7	5.0
≥ 50	11.5	4.8

TABLE 2.3   U.S. Demographic Characteristics of Smokeless Tobacco (ST) Users, by Education Level (in years), 1988

Education (in years)	% Previous ST Users	% Current ST Users
≤ 11	14.6	7.3
12	11.1	5.6
13–15	9.1	3.8
≥ 16	4.8	2.9

TABLE 2.4   U.S. Demographic Characteristics of Smokeless Tobacco (ST) Users, by Economic Level, 1988

Poverty Level	% Previous ST Users	% Current ST Users
Below	16.1	8.5
Above	9.9	4.9

TABLE 2.5   U.S. Demographic Characteristics of Smokeless Tobacco (ST) Users, by Employment Level, 1988

Employment	% Previous ST Users	% Current ST Users
Unemployed	13.0	8.3
Laborer	12.3	6.4
Blue-Collar	7.0	3.6
White-Collar	2.3	1.0

TABLE 2.6   U.S. Demographic Characteristics of Smokeless Tobacco (ST) Users, by Household Income Level, 1988

Household Income	% Previous ST Users	% Current ST Users
≤ $10,000	16.1	8.6
$10,000–29,999	4.7	2.2
≥ $30,000	3.0	1.6

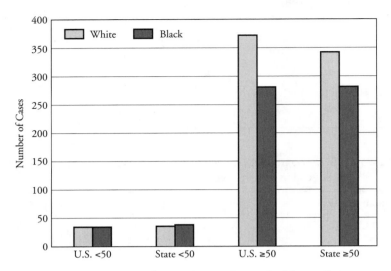

FIGURE 2.3 U.S. and State Breast Cancer Incidence Rates
per 100,000 Female Population, by Age and Race, 1988

Archie also reread the background section of a report he had prepared
a year ago for the Pershing County Department of Health. It included a
recent population profile for the state as a whole. These data showed two key
features of the state's population: (1) a large majority of the population is

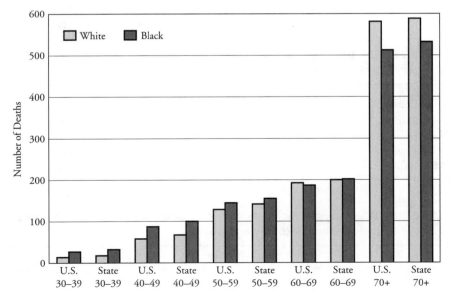

FIGURE 2.4 U.S. and State Average Breast Cancer Mortality Rates
per 100,000 Female Population, by Age and Race, 1988

TABLE 2.7   State Population, by Race, Ethnicity, and Sex, 1988

	Total Population	% of Population
Total Population	2,000,000	100.0
White males	816,000	40.8
White females	884,000	44.2
Total Whites	1,700,000	85.0
Black Males	65,600	3.3
Black Females	94,400	4.7
Total Blacks	160,000	8.0
Hispanic Males	40,400	2.0
Hispanic Females	39,600	2.0
Total Hispanics	80,000	4.0
Other Males	29,160	1.5
Other Females	30,840	1.5
Total others	60,000	3.0

White and (2) the population is very unevenly distributed by age—nearly 40 percent of the state's 2,000,000 residents are under age 20 (see Tables 2.7 and 2.8).

Identifying Gaps in the Data

In a meeting with Dr. Westphal the following week, Archie briefly summarized what he had learned and what he still needed to know about each of the two problems. For smokeless tobacco use, it was pretty clear that state rates were exceedingly high, especially among teens. This was even more troublesome considering the state's large population of people age 20 and younger. Also, smokeless tobacco appeared to be disproportionately prevalent in the most disadvantaged populations. However, these data described

TABLE 2.8   State Population, by Age and Sex, 1988

	0–19	20–39	40–59	60+	All Ages
Total males	388,073	276,787	146,479	139,821	951,160
(%)	(40.8)	(29.1)	(15.4)	(14.7)	(100.0)
Total females	389,119	293,676	196,133	169,912	1,048,840
(%)	(37.1)	(28.0)	(18.7)	(16.2)	(100.0)
Total population	784,000	542,000	368,000	306,000	2,000,000
(%)	(39.2)	(27.1)	(18.4)	(15.3)	(100.0)

only the problem behavior—smokeless tobacco use—and not its conse-quences. "I'd like to see some data showing the burden of illness and death caused by all this smokeless tobacco use," Archie said. He added, "I'd also like to see if there are any trends in smokeless tobacco use. Is it increasing? Decreasing? Staying the same?"

Archie also expressed his frustration at being unable to find out very much about breast cancer screening in the state. He told Dr. Westphal about the differences by race in breast cancer incidence and mortality, but he sensed she already knew this. "If we're really interested in screening," Archie said, "then we've got to get some mammography data. We could also use some information about trends in mammography use and breast cancer inci-dence, and it would be great if we could get some of this information by risk factors other than age—you know, like family history."

Although the data in the figures and tables provided important infor-mation about breast cancer and smokeless tobacco use, Archie realized it would be impossible to make a decision about the relative importance of each problem based on the information he had, because he had no common basis for comparing the effects of the two health problems; that is, compar-ing the level of "spit tobacco" use (a risk factor) with the incidence of breast cancer (a rate reflecting new cases of disease) seemed like comparing apples and oranges. Archie needed to find a way to compare apples with apples! Dr. Westphal agreed and suggested that Archie call the Centers for Disease Control and Prevention (CDC) and the National Center for Health Statistics (NCHS) to see what information they could provide. Those calls proved fruitful.

Filling the Gaps

Examining data on five-year trends in breast cancer mortality, Archie observed that the state rates were increasing for both Black women and White women. Changes in breast cancer mortality rates for Black women in the state were about the same as those for Black women in the United States, but rates for White women in the state appeared to be growing at a faster rate than those for U.S. White women (see Figures 2.5 and 2.6).

Archie also discovered that rates of mammography in the state were consistently lower than national averages. Within the state, fewer than 30 percent of women age 50 to 59 and fewer than a third of those age 60 to 69 had received a mammogram in the last 12 months (see Figure 2.7). Rates of mammography were lowest among those women with less than a high-school education (18.7 percent), and increased for those with more years of education (see Figure 2.8).

The fifteen-year trends in breast cancer incidence (new cases of breast cancer) were similar for the state and U.S. populations for both women

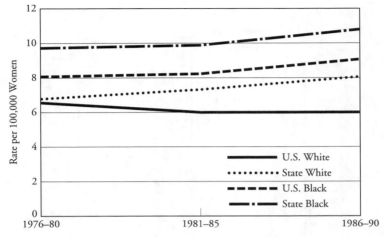

Note: Rates are five-year averages, age-adjusted to the 1970 U.S. standard population.

FIGURE 2.5   U.S. and State Fifteen-Year Trends in
Age-Adjusted* Breast Cancer Mortality Rates per 100,000
Population Age < 50, by Race, 1976–1990

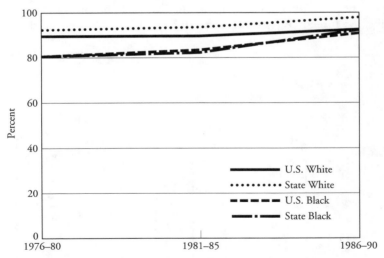

Note: Rates are five-year averages, age-adjusted to the 1970 U.S. standard population.

FIGURE 2.6   U.S. and State Fifteen-Year Trends in Age-Adjusted*
Breast Cancer Mortality Rates per 100,000 Population
Age ≥ 50, by Race, 1976–1990

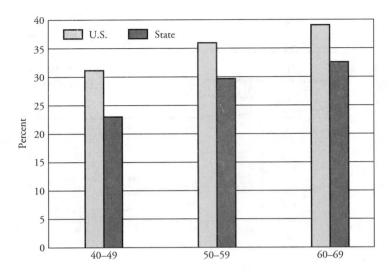

FIGURE 2.7   U.S. and State Mammography Screening Rates:
Percentages of All Women Screened, by Age, 1989

under age 50 and women 50 years or older (see Figures 2.9 and 2.10). New
cases of breast cancer among women under age 50 had increased by less than
10 percent for White women, and about 15 to 20 percent for Black women
during the fifteen-year period from 1976 to 1990. During the same time,

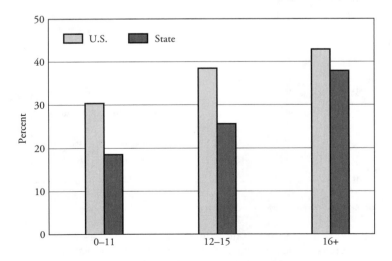

FIGURE 2.8   U.S. and State Mammography Screening Rates:
Percentages of All Women Screened, by Education Level in Years, 1989

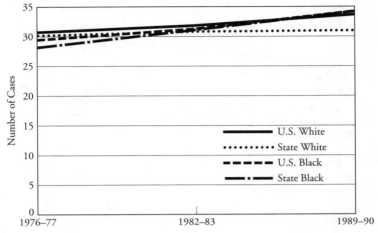

Note: Rates are two-year averages, age-adjusted to the 1970 U.S. standard population.

FIGURE 2.9   U.S. and State Fifteen-Year Trends in
Age-Adjusted* Breast Cancer Incidence Rates
per 100,000 Population Age < 50, by Race, 1976–1990

rates among both Black and White women age 50 and older had increased about 23 percent.

Archie was also able to obtain some data showing recent trends in mammography among women in the state and nationally. From 1987 to

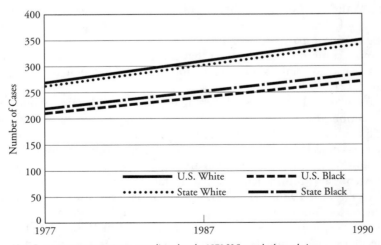

Note: Rates are two-year averages, age-adjusted to the 1970 U.S. standard population.

FIGURE 2.10   U.S. and State Fifteen-Year Trends in
Age-Adjusted* Breast Cancer Incidence Rates
per 100,000 Population Age ≥ 50, by Race, 1976–1990

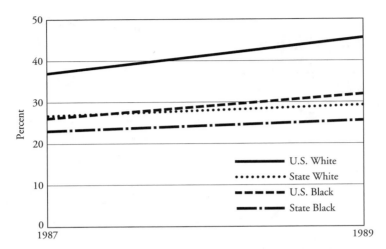

FIGURE 2.11   U.S. and State Three-Year Trends in
Mammography Screening Rates: Percentages of All Women
50 Years and Older Ever Screened, by Race, 1987–1989

1990, the proportion of women in the state who had ever received a mammogram increased by about 10 percent for both Black and White women, but this change was modest compared to national trends showing increases of nearly 20 percent for both Black and White women (see Figure 2.11).

Shifting to the new data on smokeless tobacco use, Archie saw that there were about 30,000 new cases of oral cancer each year in the United States. Although not all of these could be attributed to tobacco use, the majority of them could. He found that there were twice as many cases among men compared to women, and cancers of the mouth and pharynx were most common. Archie noted that there were relatively few oral cancer deaths per year—only about 8,000 for men and women combined (see Figure 2.12).

As he would have guessed, Archie found incidence rates of oral cancer higher among men than women. After all, he figured, they were the ones most likely to use smokeless tobacco. Overall, however, the rates were relatively low—fewer than 20 cases per 100,000 population among U.S. males, and about 6 or 7 cases per 100,000 among females (see Figure 2.13).

Archie also found data comparing rates of smokeless tobacco use in 1970 to rates for 1986. For the U.S. population, rates for chewing tobacco had increased among males age 29 and younger, but not among men in other age categories. Rates of snuff use were higher in 1986 for all but those in the oldest age groups (see Figures 2.14 and 2.15). Increases in rates of chewing tobacco and snuff use among state males were much more dramatic. For chewing tobacco use, rates nearly doubled for all males under age 39.

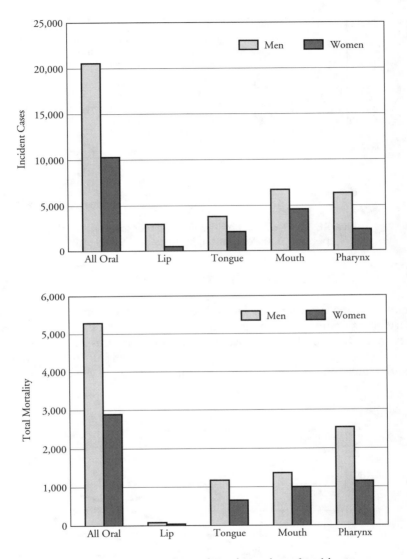

FIGURE 2.12 U.S. Estimated Total Number of Incidents
Oral Cancer Cases and Total Mortality from Oral Cancers, 1991

For snuff use, rates increased tenfold among 17-to-19-year-olds, and about sevenfold for those age 20 to 29 and 30 to 39. Even men in the 40-to-49 age category had substantially higher rates of snuff use in 1986 than in 1970 (see Figures 2.16 and 2.17).

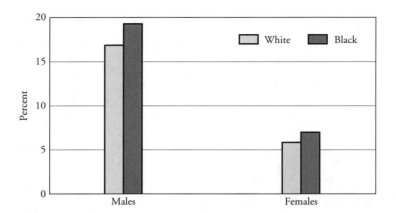

FIGURE 2.13   U.S. Estimated Oral Cancer Incidence Rates
per 100,000 Population, by Race and Sex, 1991

Weighing the Evidence

Before his next meeting with Judith Westphal, Archie prepared a brief summary of his findings, including all the relevant data tables and charts. When they met, Dr. Westphal had read his report and was pleased.

"This is good stuff, Archie. Incidentally, my son informed me that his health education teacher has told the students not to use the term smokeless

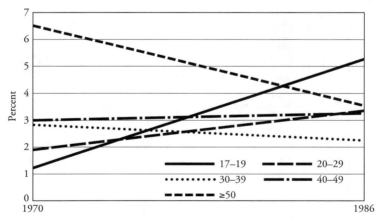

Note: More than a fourfold increase in the consumption of chewing tobacco among 17–19-year-olds between 1970 and 1986.

FIGURE 2.14   U.S. Trends (1970–1986) in Percentage of Males
Using Chewing Tobacco, by Age (by percentage who use)

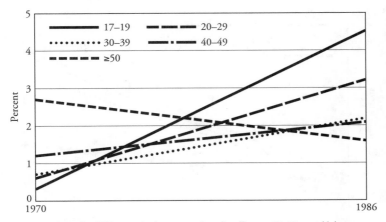

Note: More than a fourfold increase in the consumption of snuff among 17–19-year-olds between 1970 and 1986.

FIGURE 2.15   U.S. Trends (1970–1986) in Percentage of Males Using Snuff, by Age (by percentage who use)

tobacco because it leaves the impression that because it is smokeless, using it will do no harm—so do you know what they call it?"

"I do," said Archie. "Spit tobacco!"

Judith frowned. "I find it a disgusting expression."

Archie laughed. "Disgusting, but effective."

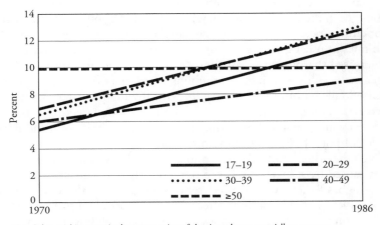

Note: Substantial increases in the consumption of chewing tobacco, especially among age groups under 40.

FIGURE 2.16   State Trends (1970–1986) in Percentage of Males Using Chewing Tobacco, by Age (by percentage who use)

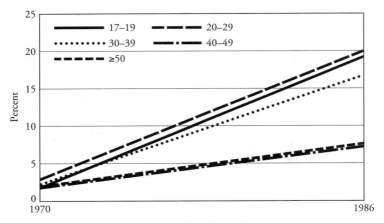

Note: Substantial increases in the consumption of snuff, especially among age groups under 40.

FIGURE 2.17   State Trends (1970–1986) in Percentage of Males Using Snuff, by Age (by percentage who use)

Archie explained that he'd had a lot of cooperation from different agencies that had provided him with data, and that many of the leads and contacts she had given him were very helpful.

Setting the report down on her desk, Judith continued, "I guess the only remaining question is which problem we go after in our proposal. What do you think, Archie? What would your recommendation be?"

Archie had expected this question and had given his answer considerable thought in the preceding few days. "Well, I think you can make a decent case for either one, really," he said. "For smokeless tobacco, we have extremely high rates of use, especially among teenagers and young men. Rates of use have increased sharply in the last fifteen years, most notably for snuff use by younger males. This is even more troubling given that 40 percent of our state population falls within the age category with the highest rates of smokeless tobacco use. There's also something appealing about targeting a problem that affects young people. Preventing diseases in teens and young adults can save a lot of potential years of life from being lost."

"On the other hand," Archie continued, "when you look at the rates of diseases caused by smokeless tobacco use—mostly oral cancers—they're just not that high. Obviously they're very serious problems for those affected, but in the big picture, they just don't affect that many people. I think we're talking about only 17 or 18 new cases per year per 100,000 population, so maybe 200 cases, tops, in our state in a year."

"As for mammography," Archie said, changing the subject, "our rates are well below national averages. Only about 30 percent of women age 50 to 59 in the state have had a mammogram in the last year, and our rates for women with less than a college education are much lower than comparable groups nationally. The trend data from the American Cancer Society show that state rates of mammography have been increasing over the last few years, but at only half the rate of increase among all women in the United States."

Archie continued. "It's weird, but even though our mammography rates are well below U.S. averages, our rates of new breast cancer cases and of breast cancer mortality are almost identical to U.S. rates. I guess maybe because we have fewer women being screened, fewer cases of breast cancer are being detected. I don't know. Would that make sense?"

Judith nodded. "Could be," she said, "but weren't incidence rates for White women in the state increasing faster than for Whites in the United States? I thought I remembered seeing that." Judith thumbed through her copy of the report, looking for the appropriate data table.

"Actually, I think you're right," Archie said. "I do remember that." Judith tapped the page when she found what she was looking for. "Here it is," she said, and gestured for Archie to continue.

"Anyway, even if our disease and death rates for breast cancer are no higher than U.S. rates, the rates are much higher than what we see for smokeless tobacco-related oral cancers. In contrast to 18 new cases of oral cancers per 100,000 people, we're talking about 300 to 350-plus cases of breast cancer among women 50 and older. It's not even close. From a public health perspective of having the greatest impact on the most people, it would be hard to choose smokeless tobacco use over mammography. So I guess that would be my recommendation. I think smokeless tobacco use is a serious problem for us, and I think we ought to try to do something about it, but I'd choose mammography for this year's new project."

Judith nodded her head in agreement. "I think you're right," she said. "These choices are always difficult ones because you'd like to be able to do something about all public health problems. You hate to say, 'this one's important and that one isn't.' But I think the data you've assembled support your decision. I would have made the same recommendation."

They decided that Archie would present his report and recommendation at the next staff meeting, and Judith would begin assembling a team to put together a program proposal for the new budget.

After Archie had presented his findings to the other staff members, Judith took over the meeting.

"Archie did a great job with these data, and that's really going to help us as we put together the background and rationale for this project," she said. "Archie, since you've already done most of the work on it, I'd like you to be responsible for writing those sections of the proposal." Archie nodded approval. Judith continued, "Now we've got to begin thinking about how we can get more women screened for breast cancer."

In the next ten minutes, Judith outlined the remaining tasks to be completed, and assigned each one to a different staff member. Elaine Elkins would identify the factors that influenced a woman's decision to seek mammography and her ongoing compliance with screening guidelines. Bill Minor would assess physicians' practice patterns as they related to breast cancer screening. Margie O'Bannon would talk to health care provider groups in the state to determine the availability and accessibility of screening services. When she was done, Judith seemed to have covered all the bases, investigating any factors that might motivate, support, or reinforce a woman's decision to seek mammography.

Four Months Later

Just as Judith Westphal had hoped, the HPCDP's new breast cancer screening initiative emerged as a top priority for the health department in its budget recommendations to the governor. The hard work of Archie Graham and other HPCDP staffers had paid off. But there was little time to celebrate. When the governor's budget bill reached the appropriations committee, the health department's proposed new initiatives became an important issue. The committee wanted further explanation of the projects, and called for testimony from the health department director, Dr. Joseph Jackson.

At 8 A.M. on the morning Dr. Jackson was scheduled to testify, his wife called the health department to tell his staff that he had been stricken with the flu and would not be able to meet with the appropriations committee as planned. Dr. Jackson asked that Judith Westphal serve in his capacity before the committee. At 8:15, Judith was informed that she was to fill in for Dr. Jackson at the 10:30 meeting at the capitol. Judith immediately contacted Archie Graham and explained that she wanted him to accompany her to the meeting for backup in the event that the committee asked questions requiring interpretation of the data upon which the breast cancer screening initiative was based.

Following Judith's testimony, the committee chair, Representative Leo Mazzone, a longtime advocate of public programs for the economically disadvantaged, questioned the importance of the new initiative.

"Dr. Westphal, thank you for taking time out of your busy day to testify before this committee," he began. "It is clear that your people have put a good deal of time and effort into this proposal." Representative Mazzone removed his glasses and rubbed his eyes before continuing. "But I must tell you, I am most curious as to how the health department can see this program as a state priority when thousands of people right under your nose, my constituents in this city, go without basic health care. Isn't it time you folks address some of the health problems that affect those in the greatest need?"

Without being combative, Judith tried to defuse Leo Mazzone's question by mentioning some of the health department programs that specifically targeted disadvantaged populations. "As for this initiative," she continued, "we believe it is a program that will benefit all women in the state. Rates of mammography in the state are lowest among minority women and women with less than a high-school education. They would stand to gain the most from this type of program." She looked over at Archie who nodded in confirmation.

Representative Mazzone asked whether the committee members had any further questions for Dr. Westphal before she was dismissed. Vard Maxwell, the most senior member of the committee, gestured to the chairman and leaned forward in his seat. He cleared his throat and sipped from a cup of water. "Mr. Chairman, this is not so much a question for Dr. Westphal as it is a comment to my colleagues on this committee," he said. "As most of you know, my wife, Nita, is a survivor of breast cancer. She's 62 years old and has lived five happy and productive years since her diagnosis and surgery. I hope and expect she's going to be around for many more, too."

He continued. "But I'm smart enough to realize that Nita's here today because she's got private insurance and a great doctor, and had regular mammograms. Her cancer was detected early when it could still be treated effectively. Not all women have that benefit. But they ought to." He eased back in his chair. "I think this is precisely the kind of program we should support." Judith smiled kindly at Representative Maxwell. Archie looked down at his notepad. The committee remained silent until the chairman spoke. "Thank you for coming today, Dr. Westphal, Mr. Graham," he said. "We appreciate your time."

Outside the room, Judith and Archie exchanged a look of pleasant surprise and walked without speaking to the elevator.

Case Analysis

Judith and Archie were fortunate that Vard Maxwell added such a compelling personal note to their presentation. However, the success of their presentation can be attributed to more than luck. Judith's sound management skills set the stage with the right questions. She anticipated the upcoming task and gave her staff enough lead time to do a thorough job. She also delegated tasks, with appropriate guidance, to Archie. Archie, in turn, used solid technical skills to obtain and analyze data, and while doing so realized that he needed some additional information in order to make an informed decision. Once he realized this, he took the initiative to pursue the missing data.

In this section, we provide some additional information and examples of how to obtain and use data—the two tasks that Judith and Archie performed so well and that are at the heart of effective public health practice.

TYPES AND SOURCES OF PUBLIC HEALTH DATA

The first step in identifying sources of information is to find out what is readily available within your organization. This may seem like an obvious suggestion, but in many large agencies (and some smaller ones, too), a wide variety of useful information sits in computers or on shelves, unbeknownst to those who might find it helpful. For example, Linda Thomas learned about the stroke belt and leading indicators of disease not from her supervisor and colleagues, but from an outside speaker!

As a first step, find out which indicators of community health status are already collected by your state and/or local health department. Annual reports, legislative testimony, and other policy documents often provide compilations of relevant data. If your health department participates in the Assessment Protocol for Excellence in Public Health (APEX/PH), you will have access to data required for a community health profile. (For a copy of APEX/PH, contact the National Association of City and County Health Officials at 202-783-5550.) APEX/PH is a workbook designed to help health department staff assess and improve their organizational capacity and work with their local communities to assess and improve health status. Several worksheets call for the following types of basic information:

- **A demographic profile** of community residents by age, sex, race/ethnicity, and socioeconomic variables (such as the percentage of the population living below the poverty level, unemployed, or receiving food stamps, WIC, or Medicaid).
- **Mortality statistics,** coded according to the *International Classification of Diseases* (discussed later), to determine the leading causes of death for each age group.

Optional data might include:

- disease prevalence by age
- leading causes of hospitalization
- perinatal indicators
- access to primary health care
- risk factors
- environmental hazards

Where can you find all this?

Mortality data are generally tracked by vital statistics departments, which also record births, marriages, and divorces. In some states, vital statistics departments are part of the health department. All 50 states collect mortality data in a standardized format, although some also capture additional information (such as smoking status). Each state's information is reported to the CDC's National Center for Health Statistics (NCHS), which compiles a national data set. (Access to national mortality data sets is discussed later.)

Mortality data sets include demographic information on the deceased, where he or she lived and died, whether or not the death occurred in a hospital or institution, and the cause of death. The cause of death is translated into a medical code described in the *Manual of the International Statistical Classification of Diseases, Injuries, and Causes of Death,* ninth revision. This is referred to as the *ICD-9 code.*

Hospital discharge data are available in 35 states and can be a useful tool for determining public health problems as well as treatment patterns, access to care, and costs associated with various diseases or procedures. Data sets typically include age, race, sex, area of residence, year of discharge, length of hospital stay, and diagnoses.

Hospital discharge data are not always found in vital statistics departments; they may be under the purview of insurance departments or governor's-level commissions. The extent to which these data are available to public health practitioners varies widely, and restrictions are common to protect individuals' privacy. Even when hospital discharge data are available, they may not cover all hospitals in a given area.

Behavioral risk factors offer important insights into the lifestyle choices that are such stubborn contributors to poor health outcomes. These are tracked through a monthly CDC telephone survey of adults, called the Behavioral Risk Factors Surveillance System (BRFSS). BRFSS is now in place in every state. For an eight- to fourteen-day period, telephone survey staff in each state conduct between 100 and 300 interviews. A set of core questions has been used consistently since the survey was introduced in 1981. The core questions cover physical activity, blood pressure, diet, body weight, smoking, alcohol consumption, and use of preventive services. The CDC also develops modules on specific topics (such as breast and cervical cancer screening or smoke detector use) that states may opt to include. States also have the option of adding state-specific questions of particular interest to them. Since 1993, the surveys have retained the core questions and rotated additional questions every year. The Youth Risk Behavior Surveillance System (YRBSS) provides similar information for high-school-age youth in the United States.

State-level data can be obtained in computer format from the CDC (see the following sections), which also compiles a national data file and related reports. Each state has a BRFSS coordinator who has access to state and national data sets, as well as CDC analyses of the data.

Two additional CDC resources can help you customize larger data sets so that they are less cumbersome. The **Health Information Retrieval System (HIRS)** allows you to specify the data sets you use most often, such as hospital databases, cancer registries, or vital records. These data sets are pretabulated so that you do not have to set them up each time you need them. Although the actual importing of data sets takes some technical skill, no programming knowledge is required once the system is set up. (For assistance or more information, contact the CDC's Office of Surveillance and Analysis at 404-488-5269.)

The CDC's **Assessment Information Manager (AIM)** provides premade templates or shells for state and local data in two areas: vital statistics and hospital discharges. Once these are loaded into the menu-driven system, a researcher with no advanced epidemiology or computer skills can retrieve, combine, and print demographic profiles, causes of mortality, perinatal indicators, years of potential life lost, and model standards. The AIM is specifically designed to support assessment processes such as APEX/PH. If data from your state's vital statistics and hospital discharge records are available in this format, for example, you could collect and track data on health objectives identified through APEX/PH or any other planning process.

Vital statistics, mortality, and hospital discharge data are just the tip of the iceberg. You should be able to find similar combinations of local-, state-, and national-level data sets for greater detail on HIV/AIDS, smoking, cardiovascular disease, specific cancers, or any other health problem. Practitioners may find Table 2.9 useful; it provides a sample of some of the major public health data sources, along with contact information. Additional information may now be available on the Internet on home pages of relevant agencies.

By definition, **national data sets** such as those described in Table 2.9 represent compilations of data submitted by states and localities. Preparing and editing data often takes months, and in some cases years, so if you are interested only in data about your state or county, you will have faster access to these types of data locally. Despite these delays, it is still worth the trouble to seek out national aggregate versions of data sets. For example, health departments in your area may already participate in data collection geared to national indicators such as *Healthy People 2000: National Health Promotion and Disease Prevention Objectives*. These types of indicators are useful for making comparisons, such as those that Archie Graham made to determine how mammography and breast cancer incidence rates in his state compared to national trends. Note that these comparisons can be made between city or county and state data as well as between local and national data.

National indicators can also help you frame the unit of measurement for a particular health problem. For example, if you were interested in improving nutrition among a particular population, what indicators would tell you that you were making progress? According to *Healthy People 2000,* you would want to track dietary fat intake, calcium intake, breast-feeding, nutrition labeling, the availability of reduced-fat processed foods, and nutrition assessments and referrals by clinicians—among many other indicators. You may also come up with additional indicators relevant to your community or program, but in any case, these can be a good starting point—especially for a disease or risk factor that is new to you.

The CDC collects, maintains, and disseminates vast amounts of health-related data. Indeed, coordinating the nation's surveillance system is one of the agency's most important and long-standing contributions to public health. Technological advances have made CDC products accessible to anyone with a computer and a modem. In addition, as described in the following sections, several products are specifically designed for public health researchers who are *not* experts in computer programming or statistical analyses.

Wide-Ranging Online Data for Epidemiologic Research (WONDER) provides on-line access to various CDC databases as well as information from other agencies. For example, through WONDER you can access data from:

- the Alcohol, Drug Abuse, and Mental Health Administration
- the Behavioral Risk Factor Surveillance System (BRFSS), maintained by the CDC
- Surveillance, Epidemiology, and End Results (SEER) data from the National Cancer Institute
- U.S. Bureau of the Census population data by age, race, sex, and county
- Disease codes from *International Classification of Diseases,* ninth revision (ICD-9) and the ICD-9 Clinical Modification
- National Hospital Discharge Survey results from the National Center for Health Statistics (NCHS), which is part of the CDC
- Underlying- and multiple-cause-of-death files from the NCHS

WONDER is menu-driven and requires no programming skills. Once you have selected the combinations of data you are seeking, you can choose different displays of information (such as tables, charts, or maps) and print these displays directly from your computer screen.

WONDER may be accessed through your local web site at: http://wonder.cdc.com.

The positive attributes of health can be defined as more than the absence of disease. Similarly, the factors that contribute to illnesses and injury are broader than strictly health-related factors. A wide range of **demographic data** can help provide a fuller picture of the determinants of health in your community. These might include data on average income levels, the number of people living below the poverty line, the unemployment rate in a given community, age distribution, race and ethnicity, Medicaid/AFDC recipients, and birth rates—among many others. Many of these indicators are derived from national census data.

Clearly, public health has moved far beyond its former confines of communicable disease control. Attention to lifestyle and behaviors as risk factors for a wide variety of diseases and conditions is just one example.

TABLE 2.9 Public Health Data Sources

Data Source	Description	For More Information, Contact . . .
Centers for Disease Control and Prevention (CDC)		
CDC Wonder/PC	A menu-driven software program providing public health professionals quick and easy access to critical data collected and analyzed by the CDC.	CDC WONDER Customer Support CDC, 1600 Clifton Road, NE, Mailstop F-51 Atlanta, GA 30333 Phone: (404) 332-4569 Fax: (770) 488-7593
CDC Information Network for Public Health Officials (INPHO)	A telecommunications network designed to link the nation's state and local health departments with the CDC. It is currently being developed in partnership with state and local public health departments, academic centers, and private foundations. The CDC recently awarded $4.3 million to twelve states (Florida, Georgia, Illinois, Indiana, Michigan, Missouri, New York, North Carolina, Oregon, Rhode Island, Washington, and West Virginia) to assist them in building their statewide information networks and information systems. INPHO will provide the public health community with ready access to the information and data needed for decision making, operation of effective programs, and timely response to public health emergencies.	Public Health Practice Program Office/ INPHO CDC Phone: (404) 639-1938
Data 2000 Monitoring System	Healthy People 2000 provides a strategy for improving the health of Americans by the end of the century through the achievement of measurable objectives and subobjectives in 22 priority areas of public health. Data 2000 is an electronic database that contains national data trends for all the HP2000 objectives and subobjectives, information about the data, and the data sources being used to track progress.	National Center for Health Statistics CDC Phone: (301) 436-3548
Behavior Risk Factor Surveillance System (BRFSS)	A national population-based telephone survey designed to assess the prevalence of health-related behavioral risk factors associated with leading causes of premature death and disability.	Behavioral Risk Factor Surveillance Branch CDC Phone: (770) 488-5292
Youth Risk Behavior Surveillance System (YRBSS)	Developed to monitor priority health risk behaviors that contribute to leading causes of mortality, morbidity, and social problems among high-school-age youth in the United States. The YRBSS provides comparable national, state, and local data and a means to monitor progress toward achieving 26 national health objectives for the year 2000.	Division of Adolescent School Health CDC Phone: (770) 488-5327

System	Description	Contact
Pediatric Nutrition Surveillance System (PedNSS)	Part of the legislatively mandated national Nutrition Monitoring System and coordinated by the CDC. The system provides nutritional status data on high-risk minority populations for state and local agency use.	Office of Maternal and Child Health CDC Phone: (770) 488-4719
Pregnancy Nutrition Surveillance System (PNSS)	Monitors nutrition-related problems and behavioral risk factors associated with low birth weight among high-risk prenatal populations.	Office of Maternal and Child Health CDC Phone: (770) 488-4719
National Notifiable Diseases Surveillance System (NNDSS)	National summaries of 40 notifiable conditions reported from 50 state health departments, New York City, Washington, D.C., and 5 U.S. territories.	Epidemiology Program Office CDC Phone: (404) 639-0080
121 Cities Weekly Mortality Surveillance System	Used by city and county health departments in 121 U.S. cities to report data on deaths from pneumonia and influenza and from all causes combined.	Systems Operations and Information Branch CDC Phone: (404) 639-3761
STD Morbidity Surveillance System	This is the national repository for STD morbidity information collected by state health departments. Summary reports of STDs are voluntarily sent to the CDC under an agreement with the Council of State and Territorial Epidemiologists.	Division of Sexually Transmitted Disease and HIV Prevention CDC Phone: (404) 639-8356
HIV Seroprevalence Surveys	The CDC has conducted standardized HIV surveys in designated subgroups of the U.S. population since 1989 as part of their effort, in collaboration with state and local health departments, other Federal agencies, blood collection agencies, and medical research institutions, to establish a surveillance system to monitor the HIV epidemic in the United States.	Division of HIV/AIDS CDC Phone: (404) 639-2090
Surveillance and Evaluation of Blood Donors for HIV	This system reports data to the CDC on individual blood donors testing positive for HIV antibodies. Data are collected from the routine testing of blood at blood donor centers.	Seroepidemiology Branch, Division of HIV/AIDS CDC Phone: (404) 639-2080

continued

TABLE 2.9 *continued*

Data Source	Description	For More Information, Contact . . .
Birth Defects Monitoring Program (BDMP)	A national hospital-based surveillance system for birth defects. The data are analyzed to identify unusual trends and geographic differences that may signal the presence of environmental or other risk factors for birth defects.	Birth Defects and Genetic Diseases CDC Phone: (770) 488-7160
CDC National Center for Health Statistics (NCHS)		
National Health Interview Survey (NHIS)	A continuing nationwide household interview survey that has been conducted since 1957. Data are used to provide national estimates on the incidence of acute illness and injuries, the prevalence of chronic conditions and impairments, the extent of disability, the utilization of health care services, and other health-related topics.	Division of Health Interview Statistics NCHS Phone: (301) 436-7089
National Health and Nutrition Examination Survey (NHANES)	NCHS has conducted seven national examination surveys of the U.S. population since 1960. The most recent survey, NHANES III, was conducted between 1988 and 1994. The surveys are designed to produce information on the health status of the nation and regions of the country. State or local information is generally not available except through inference from the national data. The data from these studies have been used to estimate the prevalence of diseases, risk factors, and conditions as well as to produce national reference distributions and estimate secular changes in health status, health programs, and unmet needs of health care.	Division of Health Examinations and Statistics NCHS Phone: (301) 436-7068, ext. 123
National Maternal and Infant Health Survey	Presents data from the 1991 longitudinal survey, which was a follow-up of the women interviewed for the 1988 National Maternal and Infant Health Survey. The purpose of the 1988 survey was to study factors related to poor pregnancy outcomes (*i.e.*, fetal and infant loss and low birth weight).	Division of Vital Statistics NCHS Phone: (301) 436-8951
National Survey of Family Growth	This survey is to examine the variables that affect the nation's birthrate, including contraception, sterilization, infertility, and maternal and infant health topics such as prenatal care and breast feeding.	Office of Family Growth NCHS Phone: (301) 436-8731

Hard Copy Data for NCHS	Data from the surveys and studies conducted by NCHS are presented in a variety of publications. Many of the reports are part of the Vital and Health Statistics series, which now includes more than 900 individual publications grouped into several subseries.	Data Dissemination Branch Division of Data Services, NCHS 6525 Belcrest Road Hyattsville, MD 20782 Phone: (301) 436-8500

Health Care Financing Administration (HCFA)

State Profile Data System (spDATA)	Contains selected characteristics from Medicaid, state plans, pending state plan amendments (SPA), and supplementary information submitted with SPAs. It is not an automated database for the entire state plan, nor does it automate the state plan process. SPAs are entered as separate records so that the user can examine state plans with effective dates of 10/1/91 to close of business yesterday.	For a copy of a report, contact: Phone: (410) 966-3341 For questions about the content of spDATA, contact: Phone: (410) 966-5935
Medicaid Statistical Information System (MSIS) and State Medicaid Research Files (SMRF)	The purpose of MSIS and SMRF is to collect, manage, analyze, and disseminate information on eligible recipients, utilization, and payment for services covered by state Medicaid programs. Participation is voluntary.	For MSIS, contact: HCFA Phone: (410) 597-3903 For SMRFs, contact: HCFA Phone: (410) 597-3892
Medicaid Statistics: Program and Financial Statistics	This publication summarizes program and financial Medicaid statistics on a national, regional, and state-by-state basis. Charts and tables contained in this book are collected from state-reported characteristic data and actual federal outlays of Medicaid expenditures.	Medicaid Bureau, HCFA Phone: (410) 966-3397

continued

TABLE 2.9 *continued*

Data Source	Description	For More Information, Contact . . .
Agency for Health Care Policy and Research (AHCPR)		
Health Care Cost and Utilization Project	HCUP-3 has four broad objectives: to obtain data primarily from statewide information sources, specifically state agencies and private data organizations; to design and develop a multistate health care database containing information on hospitals and their patients, to be used for health services research and health policy analysis; to use these data to conduct research on cost and quality of health services; and to design versions of the data that can be shared with a broad set of public and private users.	Center for Intramural Research AHCPR Phone: (301) 594-1410
National Medical Expenditure Survey	A series of surveys providing extensive information on health expenditures by or on behalf of American families and individuals, the financing of these expenditures, and each person's use of services. The survey has two components: institutional and household. The two surveys yield comprehensive population-based estimates that permit separate and comparative analyses of most population groups of policy interest.	Center for Intramural Research AHCPR Phone: (301) 594-1400
AIDS Cost and Services Utilization Survey	A longitudinal study of persons with HIV-related disease that uses a combination of personal interviews and abstraction of medical and billing records. Results allow for an examination of a wide range of issues, including patterns of use of medical and nonmedical services, expenditures for medical services, the relationship between use and source of payment for care, and changes in these factors over the course of the illness that can be analyzed for HIV-infected persons receiving care from major providers located in large urban centers.	Center for Research, Dissemination and Liaison AHCPR Phone: (301) 594-1354, ext. 117
National Institutes of Health		
National Library of Medicine: National Information Center on Health Services Research and Health Care Technology (NICHSR)	The goals of NICHSR are to make results of health services, research, including practice guidelines and technology assessments, readily available to the professionals who serve these groups; to improve access to information needed by the creators of health services research; and to contribute to the information infrastructure needed to foster patient record systems that can produce useful health services research data as a by-product of providing health care.	Office of Health Services Research Information National Library of Medicine Phone: (310) 496-0176

National Cancer Institute:
Surveillance, Epidemiology, and End Results (SEER)

Collects data on a routine basis from designated population-based cancer registries in various areas of the country. Trends in cancer incidence, mortality, and patient survival in the United States, as well as many other studies, are derived from this data bank.

SEER Program
NCI/DCPC/SP
Cancer Statistics Branch, EPN 343 J
9000 Rockville Pike
Bethesda, MD 20892
Phone: (301) 402-0816

National Institute on Drug Abuse:
National Pregnancy and Health Survey

The first nationally representative survey on the prevalence of drug use among women who give birth in the United States. It is a one-time survey of a representative sample of women delivering live infants in hospitals in the United States. Data were collected for 1992.

Div. of Epidemiology & Prevention Research, NIDA
Phone: (301) 443-6637

Press Office, NIDA
Phone: (301) 443-6245

National Institute on Drug Abuse:
Drug Abuse Treatment Outcome Study (DATOS)

A multifaceted, multiyear investigation of treatment effectiveness based on a nation-wide purposeful sample of short- and long-term methadone maintenance, short- and long-term residential treatment, and outpatient drug-free programs. The sample consists of 12,000 individuals entering one or more of 100 drug-abuse treatment programs over a two-year period. A sample of 4,500 individuals were interviewed after leaving their respective treatment programs. Included with the overall DATOS family of database is (1) the DATOS of Adolescents (DATOS-A), a longitudinal prospective study of drug abuse treatment effectiveness in the adolescent population based on a sample of outpatient and residential treatment programs, and (2) the Early Retrospective Study of Cocaine Treatment Outcomes, an accelerated two-year retrospective study of a sample of treatment program records and a follow-up interview of clients from between eight and twelve program sites participating in DATOS.

Phone: (301) 443-4060

continued

TABLE 2.9 *continued*

Data Source	Description	For More Information, Contact . . .
National Institute on Alcohol, Alcoholism, and Alcohol Abuse: National Longitudinal Alcohol Epidemiologic Survey (NLAES)	The purpose of this survey is to determine the prevalence, incidence, remission, chronicity, and stability rates of various drinking levels, alcohol-use disorders, and their associated disabilities, including simultaneous and concurrent substance use patterns. NLAES also provides information on alcohol and drug treatment utilization among persons in the general population as well as data concerning access and barriers to alcohol-related treatment services, particularly among low-income groups, women, young adults, and minorities. It provides data on the number of people in the population in need of but not currently receiving treatment as well as individual awareness concerning warning label information contained on alcoholic beverage containers. The survey also identifies risk factors that initiate and/or maintain various drinking levels, alcohol-use disorders, and their associated disabilities.	Division of Biometry and Epidemiology NIAAA Phone: (301) 443-3306
National Institute on Mental Health: Epidemiologic Catchment Area Program and National Comorbidity Study	The purpose of this study is to assess the prevalence and incidence of specific mental and addictive disorders, to estimate rates of health and mental-health services use, to study factors influencing the development and continuance of disorders, and to study factors influencing use of services.	ECA, National Institute on Mental Health Phone: (301) 443-3774 Institute for Social Research/Survey Research Center The University of Michigan Phone: (313) 936-0550

Substance Abuse and Mental Health Service Administration

Data Source	Description	For More Information, Contact . . .
Office of Applied Studies: National Household Survey on Drug Abuse	The primary source of statistical information on the use of illegal drugs by the U.S. population. Since 1971, the survey has collected data by means of a questionnaire to a representative sample of the noninstitutionalized population, twelve years of age and older, at their places of residence. The primary purpose of this survey is to provide estimates of the incidence, prevalence, consequences, and patterns of drug use and abuse, including alcohol and tobacco. The questionnaire is designed to provide estimates of lifetime, previous, and current (in the past year) drug use, frequency of use, problems associated with use, and attitudes about drug use. The data help identify the groups most at risk for illicit drug use and the drugs that are most commonly used.	Office of Applied Studies SAMHSA Phone: (301) 443-0021

Office of Applied Studies: State Alcohol and Drug Abuse Profile (SADAP)	An annual survey of state alcohol- and drug-abuse agencies, conducted by the National Association of State Alcohol and Drug Abuse Directors since 1982. The information is derived from data voluntarily submitted by the states. The overall purpose of the profile is to provide information on various aspects of the field of alcohol and other drug abuse (AODA) prevention, make state comparisons, and identify innovative services and programs in other states.	NASADAD Phone: (202) 783-6868
Center for Substance Abuse Treatment: State Systems Development Program (SSDP)	A comprehensive, systematic approach to administering the Substance Abuse Prevention and Treatment Block Grant. It has six components: data collection from the Substance Abuse Prevention and Treatment Block Grant application; State Needs Assessments Studies: State Technical Reviews; State Technical Assistance; Treatment Improvement Protocols; and State Information Systems.	Information Services and Analysis Branch Division of State Programs Center for Substance Abuse Treatment SAMHSA Phone: (301) 443-7747
Center for Mental Health Services: National Reporting Program for Mental Health Statistics (NRP)	Collects national statistics on specialty mental health organizations and the people served by such organizations. Three data-collection efforts are conducted by the NRP: Inventory of Mental Health Organizations and General Hospital Mental Health Services; Annual Census of Patient Characteristics in State and County Mental Hospitals; and Sample Surveys of Clients/Patients in Mental Health Organizations and General Hospital Psychiatric Services.	CMHS, SAMHSA Phone: (301) 443-3343

Source: *A Compendium of Selected Public Health Data Sources.* Prepared by Walcoff & Associates, Inc., for the Agency for Health Care Policy and Research, December 1994.

Indeed, public health's dual focus on individual and community health brings an even wider scope of problems into focus, many of which may not be traditionally thought of as health related. For example, in most communities, violence and motor vehicle injuries are heavy contributors to morbidity and mortality. Understanding their toll on communities and designing interventions to reduce that toll requires interaction with numerous other agencies: law enforcement, criminal justice, education, and traffic safety, among others.

These agencies offer combinations of national, state, and local data sets that are comparable to those for health indicators discussed earlier. For example, the National Highway Traffic Safety Administration maintains the Fatal Accident Reporting System (FARS), which is based on state and local data reported from police investigations of automobile crash sites. The National Institute of Justice maintains a drugs and crime data center that provides statistics and publications (800-666-3332).

In short, for any given health-related problem that is not only within your community health department's purview, follow the trail from the local level up to state and national agencies. Eventually, you will encounter a database!

Last but not least, **human beings** are a tremendous source of information and insight. Databases are useful but do not capture the cumulative wisdom and interpretation skills that reside in an experienced mind. For example, Judith Westphal helped streamline Archie Graham's search, even though he was familiar with the relevant data sets and obtained good information on his own.

Talk to people in your agency and outside of it. Participate actively in a professional association. Read what they send you. Call up authors of articles. If they don't have time to talk to you, they will tell you so, and you will be no worse off. However, you do owe your interview subjects the courtesy of some preparation and thinking ahead of time; it is not their job to teach you Breast Cancer 101.

A CAUTIONARY NOTE

Within reason, a variety of different sources and portrayals of information will help you develop a richer, more nuanced description of the problem. Data on public health problems reflect the complexity and interrelated nature of the problems themselves. We rarely see a clean, unbroken line between cause and effect, nor do we have the luxury of a recent survey polling the exact population we're interested in about the exact behavior we want to modify. Instead, we find ourselves trying to disentangle a knot of behaviors, socioeconomic conditions, susceptibility to disease, and sheer chance. Some data may contradict each other, or fall short in terms of comprehensiveness, or seem out of date—among many other drawbacks.

These data problems don't necessarily have to be solved, but they do have to be acknowledged in your assumptions and in your portrayals and uses of data. For example, we don't know the true homeless population in the community because, among other census problems, estimates cannot capture the number of people who are doubled up in friends' and relatives' apartments because they cannot afford their own. When we explain why we have designed a health care program for the homeless based on larger estimates of need than the documented homeless population, this is one of the reasons. As you inform yourself about the health problem you are trying to address, keep track of gaps in your data and how they affect your intervention and its evaluation.

USING PUBLIC HEALTH DATA

Recall that Archie Graham and Judith Westphal had a definite purpose in mind in collecting their data. Their research, analysis, and recommendations on behalf of a particular program reflect a critical use of data: choosing among competing public health priorities.

The Massachusetts Department of Health has developed a community health decision-making matrix that is similar to the steps followed by Archie and Judith.[3] For each community health problem you are considering, ask the following four sets of questions:

1. **Priority**
   - Do members of the community agree that this health problem is a priority?

2. **Data Availability**
   - Do direct indicators of this health problem exist?
   - Do indicators of risk behaviors related to this health problem exist?
   - Are direct indicators or indicators of related risk behaviors readily available elsewhere?
   - Are they available at the community level?

3. **Scope**
   - Does this health problem exist to a sufficient extent to warrant consideration (number of cases, crude rate, age-adjusted rate)?
   - What is the impact of this health problem in this community, relative to the country, the state, or other communities?
   - What is the impact of this health problem relative to other health problems?
   - What is the impact of this health problem for one group compared to other groups?
   - What is the dollar burden of this health problem?

4. Possibility of Successful Intervention

- Is this health problem preventable?
- Is this health problem treatable?
- Are resources available to intervene in this health problem?
- Is improvement in this health problem possible?
- Is intervention in this health problem cost effective, relative to other interventions?

Two specific examples from North Carolina and Oregon show how answering these types of questions can yield useful tools for describing the problem and for motivating action.

The North Carolina Report Card

The 1995 North Carolina Report Card for the state's Child Health Day (Figure 2.18) was prepared by the North Carolina Institute of Medicine in collaboration with the Division of Maternal and Child Health within the Department of Environment, Health and Natural Resources; the North Carolina Pediatric Society; and the state's Area Health Education Centers. The report card's authors selected health indicators in nineteen categories relevant to the health of children and adolescents, ranging from child abuse and maltreatment to teen pregnancies, injuries, and immunization rates. For each indicator, the report card shows where North Carolina stood in 1993 or 1994 (the most recent years for which data were available), and how these compared to state and/or national goals for the year 2000. Grades were assigned for each indicator, depending on the size of the gap between current indicators and the year 2000 goals. The overall message from these comparisons is prominently displayed on the front cover of the report card: "C-minus—We can do better!"

Oregon's Benchmarks

Oregon's Benchmarks are standards for measuring statewide progress and government performance, and form the basis for reporting to the state legislature. First published in 1991 after a statewide strategic planning effort and a series of community meetings and debates, the benchmarks are intended to foster consensus about which goals are important, and why. In addition to health benchmarks, the process includes benchmarks for education, the environment, and the economy. Most significantly, the benchmarks are designed to measure results and outcomes rather than inputs. This means that instead of only measuring the dollars spent on a program or counting the number of times a service has been provided, state agencies must measure and report on the outcomes of these activities.

1995
North Carolina
Report Card

CHILD HEALTH DAY

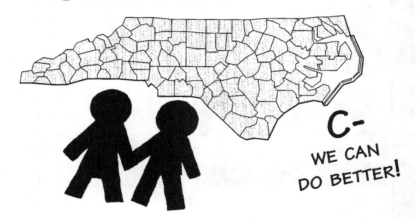

C-
WE CAN
DO BETTER!

OCTOBER 2nd

NORTH CAROLINA INSTITUTE OF MEDICINE
Citizens dedicated to improving the health of North Carolinians

DEHNR
NC Division of Maternal & Child Health,
Department of Environment, Health
and Natural Resources

NORTH CAROLINA
PEDIATRIC SOCIETY

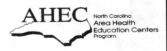
AHEC
North Carolina
Area Health
Education Centers
Program

In collaboration with The American Health Foundation, New York, NY

FIGURE 2.18 North Carolina Child Health Report Card

(figure continues through page 56)

HEALTH INDICATOR:	Year	NC Data	Target for Year 2000[16,17]	Grade
Alcohol, Tobacco and Substance Abuse				
Cigarette Smoking				
% daily smokers, grades 11-12[1]	1993	21.0	NC Goal: 9.0	D
Smokeless Tobacco Use				
% using in past 30 days, grades 11-12[1]	1993	11.7	NC Goal: 4.0	D
Marijuana Use				
% using in past 30 days, grades 11-12[1]	1993	15.0	NC Goal: 8.0	D
Alcohol				
% of students grades 11-12 who drank beer in past 30 days[1]	1993	44.0	NC Goal: 17.0	D
Cocaine				
% of students who said they used in past month[2]	1993	2.0		D
Asthma				
# of hospital discharges per 10,000 population, ages 0-14[3]	1992	24.5	US Goal: less than 30 per 10,000	A
Child Abuse and Maltreatment				
Number of cases[4]	1994	18,397	NC Goal: 22,274	B-
Child Sexual Abuse				
Number of cases[1]	1993	1,447	NC Goal: 1,365	B-
Communicable Diseases				
# of syphilis, gonorrhea, chlamydia cases, ages 15-24[1]	1993	28,407	NC Goal: 23,968	B-
# of reported cases of children, ages 0-9, with AIDS[5]	1993	7		C

HEALTH INDICATOR:	Year	NC Data	Target for Year 2000[16,17]	Grade
Immunization Rates				
% of children under 2 years with basic series completed[6]	1991	64.9	NC Goal: 90.0	B-
% of children with basic series completed at school entry[6]	1994	98	NC Goal: 98.0	A
Vaccine-Preventable Diseases (# cases ages 0-19)[7]				
Measles	1994	3	US Goal: 0	A-
Mumps	1994	73	US Goal: 0	C
Rubella	1994	0	US Goal: 0	A
Diphtheria	1994	0	US Goal: 0	A
Pertussis	1994	140	US Goal: 1,000 cases	C
Tetanus	1994	0	US Goal: 0	A
Polio	1994	0	US Goal: 0	A
Hepatitis B, # of cases per 100,000 population	1994	4.1	US Goal: 9.4	A
Hemophilus influenza, Type B	1994	32		B
Dental Disease				
Sealants: % of children with one or more sealants, 5th and 6th graders[8]	1994	23	NC Goal: 50; US Goal: 50	C-
% of children on fluoridated water systems[8]	1994	78		C+
Environmental Health				
% of preschool children screened for lead levels[9]	1994	15	NC Goal: 40.0	D
% of screened children with elevated blood lead ($\geq$15μg/dl), ages 6 months to 6 years[9]	10/92-9/94	2.5	US Goal: 2.0	C
Head Start				
% of eligible 3 and 4 year olds enrolled[10]	1994-95	31.9		C

FIGURE 2.18 *continued*

HEALTH INDICATOR:	Year	NC Data	Target for Year 2000[16,17]	Grade
Injuries				
Unintentional				
Motor vehicle death rate, ages 15-24[1]	1991-93	33.6	NC Goal: 29.6	C
# of drowning deaths, ages 0-19[14]	1993	56		C
Fires/Burns, # of deaths, ages 0-19[14]	1993	20		C
Poisoning, # of deaths, ages 0-19[14]	1993	4		C
Intentional (# of deaths)				
Suicide, ages 0-19[14]	1993	61		C -
Homicide, ages 0-19[14]	1993	135		C -
Firearms, ages 0-19[14]	1993	161		C -
Early intervention to reduce effects of developmental delay, emotional disturbance, and/or chronic illness[15]	1994	6,104	NC Goal: 8,000	B
Nutrition[1]				
% Overweight:				
Low income children ages 0-4	1992	7.1	NC Goal: 5.0	C
Low income children ages 5-11	1992	17.1	NC Goal: 10.0	D
Persons 12-19	1992	40	NC Goal: 15.0; US Goal: 15.0	D
Physical Fitness[2]				
% of all high school students with physical education classes during an average school week	1993	47		C

HEALTH INDICATOR:	Year	NC Data	Target for Year 2000[16,17]	Grade
Infant Mortality[11]				
Total # deaths/1,000 live births	1994	10.0	NC Goal: 7.4; US Goal: 7.0	C
Non-white	1994	15.6	NC Goal: 8.7 US Goal for African Americans: 11.0	D
% Low Birth Weight (5.5 lbs. or less)[11]				
Total	1994	8.7	NC Goal: 7.0; US Goal: 5.0	B
Non-White	1994	13.1	NC Goal: 10.4 US Goal for African Americans: 9.0	C
Teen Pregnancies (ages 15-17/1,000 girls in age group)[1]				
Total	1993	62.4	NC Goal: 63.0 US Goal: 50	A -
Non-White	1993	110.7	NC Goal: 86.7	B -
Prenatal Care (% of mothers aged 10-19 having LATE or NO PRENATAL CARE)[12]				
Total	1988-92	44.5		C
White	1988-92	37.1		C
Minorities	1988-92	52.3		D+
% of Live Births with NO PRENATAL CARE, Mothers' Ages 10-17[13]				
Total	1992	2.9		C
White	1992	1.9		C
Non-White	1992	3.7		C

FIGURE 2.18 *continued*

References for Child Health Report Card: October 2, 1995

[1]Blue KP. Charting the Course: North Carolina's Progress Towards the Healthy Carolinians 2000 Objectives. CHES Studies, The State Center for Health and Environmental Statistics, DEHNR, November 1994.

[2]State Center for Health and Environmental Statistics. North Carolina Adolescent Health Facts: Personal Health Habits. DEHNR, January 1995.

[3]NC Medical Database Commission. Analysis by the Cecil G. Sheps Center for Health Services Research, UNC-CH, of Oct. 1992-Sept. 1993 patient origin data for admissions of ages 0-14 with primary diagnosis 493 (asthma), August 1995.

[4]NC Division of Social Services. Central Registry Reports of Child Abuse and Neglect, 1994.

[5]Surles KB. The Health of Young Children in North Carolina: Recent Trends and Patterns. CHES Studies, The State Center for Health and Environmental Statistics, DEHNR, May 1995.

[6]NC Division of Maternal and Child Health, DEHNR, 1995.

[7]Data provided by the State Center for Health and Environmental Statistics, DEHNR, September 1995.

[8]NC Division of Dental Health, DEHNR, 1995.

[9]NC Division of Environmental Health, DEHNR, August 1995.

[10]NC Child Advocacy Institute. Early Childhood Index. Raleigh, NC, March 1995.

[11]CHES Studies, The State Center for Health and Environmental Statistics, DEHNR, August 1995.

[12]Surles KB. Adolescent Health in North Carolina: The Last 15 Years. CHES Studies, The State Center for Health and Environmental Statistics, DEHNR, January 1995.

[13]Guild PA, Schectman R, Musselman D. Consensus in Region IV: Maternal and Infant Health and Family Planning Indicators for Planning and Assessment. Region IV Network for Data Management and Utilization. Cecil G. Sheps Center for Health Services Research, University of North Carolina at Chapel Hill, September 1994.

[14]NC Detailed Mortality Statistics – 1993, The State Center for Health and Environmental Statistics, DEHNR, November 1994.

[15]North Carolina Interagency Coordinating Council. Annual Report, 1994.

[16]Healthy Carolinians 2000. The Report of the Governor's Task Force on Health Objectives for the Year 2000, November 1992.

[17]Healthy People 2000: National Health Promotion and Disease Prevention Objectives. US Department of Health and Human Services, Public Health Service, DHHS Publication No. (PHS)91-50212, 1991.

Data for this Report Card were compiled by Jane T. Kolimaga, M.A., Associate Director for Planning and Policy Analysis; design and layout were done by Diana N. Osborne, B.A., Information and Communication Specialist, both of the Cecil G. Sheps Center for Health Services Research, University of North Carolina at Chapel Hill.

FIGURE 2.18   *continued*

Because it covers so many different topics, the Oregon benchmarks process quickly yielded a large number of objectives for state programs—272 of them, to be exact. To help direct resources to the most pressing problems in the state, the list was divided into *urgent* and *core* benchmarks. Urgent benchmarks are those that are leading indicators of other benchmarks and must be addressed within the next several years. If progress is not made in addressing the urgent benchmarks, progress in these and other areas could be jeopardized in the future. For example, preventing teen pregnancy, improving early childhood cognitive and social development, and increasing access to health care (especially in rural areas) are defined as urgent benchmarks because of their impact on other health and quality-of-life issues. A sample page from Oregon's Student Health Benchmarks is shown in Figure 2.19.

Student Health

Health Practices and Fitness

	1970	1980	1990	1992	1995	2000	2010
29. Percentage of students free of involvement with alcohol in the previous month							
a. Eighth grade			77%	74%	92%	98%	99%
b. Eleventh grade			56%	63%	75%	85%	90%
30. Percentage of students free of involvement with illicit drugs in the previous month							
a. Eighth grade			86%	89%	95%	99%	99%
b. Eleventh grade			77%	80%	85%	98%	99%
31. Percentage of students free of involvement with tobacco in the previous month							
a. Eighth grade			87%	85%	95%	95%	99%
b. Eleventh grade			77%	81%	85%	95%	99%
32. Sexually transmitted disease rate per 10,000 Oregonians ages 10–19			89.7	92.5	75.0	50.0	20.0
33. Percentage of students who carry weapons to school							
34. Percentage of children in grades 9–12 who exercise aerobically at least three times per week				74%	80%	90%	99%

High-School to Post-Secondary Educational Attainment

Current Transitions from Secondary Education

	1970	1980	1990	1992	1995	2000	2010
35. Percentage of high-school students with significant involvement in professional-technical education and entrepreneurial programs		7%	9%	9%	18%	35%	55%
36. Percentage of high-school students enrolled in structured work-experience programs			3%	3%	18%	35%	55%
37. Percentage of disabled high-school students moving directly from high school to competitive or supported employment				5%	15%	50%	80%
38. High-school graduation rate			73%	76%	83%	93%	95%

Figure 2.19   Oregon Student Health Benchmarks (page 31)

MANAGED-CARE ORGANIZATIONS

Both the North Carolina and Oregon examples reflect a trend toward monitoring health outcomes and using them to provide a rationale for how resources are allocated. This is occurring not only in public health, but in the private health sector as well, largely due to the spread of managed care as a means of financing and offering health care.

The term *managed care* describes different arrangements among individual health care consumers, providers, insurers, and purchasers (particularly those who purchase on a large scale, such as employers or government entities). Initially fueled by the cost-containment interests of private employers, the explosive growth in managed care is affecting health care delivery in both the private and public sectors throughout the United States. Currently, 90 million Americans with private insurance are enrolled in some type of managed-care organization (MCO), along with one-third of low-income Medicaid recipients who receive health care from the government, and 10 percent of elderly Medicare recipients.

The features and effects of managed care vary from state to state and community to community, but enrollment is generally growing across the country. In terms of community health promotion, the rapid growth of managed care has several important implications. One implication of the pressure to keep medical costs down is the increased attention given to prevention as part of routine health care, such as coverage for routine screening exams. Similarly, competitive and regulatory forces now create incentives for managed-care organizations to monitor and document the kinds of indicators of community health—such as immunization rates—that used to be tracked exclusively by public health agencies.

A key data source about managed care and health status is generated by the Health Plan Employer Data and Information Set (HEDIS), which is administered by the National Committee for Quality Assurance (NCQA). The NCQA is a national organization representing consumers, purchasers, and providers of managed health care. It accredits quality-assurance programs in managed-care organizations and coordinates programs for assessing the quality of care throughout the industry. The latest version of HEDIS includes 75 measures to track whether health plans affect the health status of enrolled members, how effectively they address specific health problems (such as cancer, heart disease, smoking, and diabetes), and whether consumers are satisfied with the care they receive. The latest version of HEDIS not only includes numerous indicators relevant to prevention, but also combines private and public health data by including Medicare and Medicaid data.

As these examples show, effective community health promotion is built on a foundation of relevant, useful data. Getting the right data is only half the battle. As Judith Westphal and Archie Graham demonstrated, asking the right questions before, during, and even after the data collection process is critical to streamlining the search. Although the data collection and analysis process is time-consuming and can be frustrating, solid preparation and defensible choices yield the most gratifying returns: consensus about priorities and the resolve to move forward in addressing them.

SUMMARY

In this chapter, we have tried to point out that health-related data constitute a critical source of knowledge for planners. For the most part, the data are readily available and accessible to those responsible for planning health promotion programs. We have found that effective health promotion practioners seem to operate on three assumptions about health-related data:

1. In the absence of relevant data about the health of the population we serve, we cannot set priorities, plan programs with precision, or determine how or whether those programs work.
2. We must know what questions to ask before, during, and even after the data-collection process.
3. Human beings are an essential source of information, and their opinions and views should be integrated into all health promotion program decisions.

We have used numerous examples of data in this chapter to familiarize readers with the vast health information sources available and accessible in the field. In so doing, we recognize that some may interpret this to be akin to data collection "overkill." Our position is simply this: Responsible planners need to be aware of where the data sources are and how to inquire about the relevance of those data to their various health promotion tasks. Somewhere between the extremes of operating on intuition and no information on the one hand, and the paralysis that results from having mounds of data on the other lies the prudent middle ground.

ENDNOTES

1. While our description follows the general process used by states in the United States, many of the same principles hold for provinces, states, and territories in other nations.
2. Terms referencing ethnicity continue to be a source of considerable discussion and debate. In this case story, we have chosen to use the term "Black" rather than "African-American" because the data do not enable us to make the distinction between people of black color who may not be African.
3. *Health Status Indicators: Community Health Network Areas.* Massachusetts Department of Public Health. Boston: June 1994.

CHAPTER 3

Discovering the Causes

Case Story
WHAT CAUSES THE CAUSES?

Forty tables, six places at each one: not an empty seat in the house. The tables were covered with starched white cloths, each one topped with two candles and a bouquet of freshly cut flowers. A portable podium centered on a small platform stood at one end of the room, and behind it hung a gold banner with blue letters that read: "Our Kids Count." The sounds of dinner-table conversation were complemented by the almost unnoticeable background strains of highbrow elevator music. But all the ambience, including the servers decked out in black and white, could not camouflage the fact that this was the Whitehall Junior High multipurpose room!

The general manager of the new Marriott Hotel had offered the use of one of the hotel's ballrooms at no charge, but the planning committee insisted that the site of the banquet honoring the *Our Kids Count Coalition* volunteers should be held at the site where it had all started five years ago.

* * *

In March 1990, a small group of parents decided to tackle the problem of underage drinking and drug use. They called themselves Villagers Who Care, after the African proverb, "It takes an entire village to raise a child." They joined forces with the Whitehall YMCA, the YWCA, the PTA, and the local cooperative extension office. This new alliance took on the name The Our Kids Count Coalition. Their goal was to plan and sponsor a community workshop on the problem of substance abuse among kids. The workshop was held in the junior high school's multipurpose room and drew 115 participants. The meeting, which lasted 2½ hours, was coordinated by Rachel Warren, the leader of Villagers Who Care. In the first hour, participants heard two speakers. One was an evaluation specialist from the state department of education, who presented data comparing national patterns of alcohol, tobacco, and drug use over the past five years with trends seen in the Whitehall area over the same five-year period.

The second presenter was Dr. Dick Loman, a professor of health education and behavioral science at State University, who described the educa-

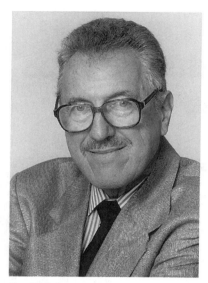

Dr. Dick Loman

tional, behavioral, and social factors that are usually associated with higher rates of substance abuse. Rachel and others were particularly impressed by the clarity and logic of Dr. Loman's presentation. The remaining hour and a half was dedicated to questions, comments, and discussion.

During the four years that followed that first meeting, Dick Loman had played a key role in the development and implementation of the intervention programs supported by the Our Kids Count Coalition.

*   *   *

With few people noticing, Mayor Carl Crawford walked over to the podium. The room quieted as he tapped a spoon against his water glass. He then tapped the microphone with his finger and asked, "Is this working?"

"Yes," the audience responded.

"Evenings like this one make my job worth doing."

A friendly heckler shouted, "Please, no speeches tonight, Mr. Mayor!"

Carl laughed. "Not a chance. I want to thank you all for taking the time and effort to join in this celebration. It is inspiring to see this kind of community commitment. At this time, I want to turn the podium over to the champion and president of the Our Kids Count Coalition, Rachel Warren."

The applause was instant, heartfelt, and long. Rachel was simultaneously proud and embarrassed.

As she approached the podium, she raised a small booklet and said, "I want to read a passage from this report. It is the 1995 annual report of the task force on substance abuse from our neighboring state, Ohio."

> It is probably true that drug dealing and alcohol abuse in suburbia is less likely to occur in plain sight, or to cause the neighborhood blight seen in some inner cities. But it is, nevertheless, there. It is hidden, and because it is hidden, it is more insidious. Families with resources and power can harbor secrets about substance abuse that contribute to shame and denial that leads to resistance to action by schools, religious leaders, and sometimes law enforcement.

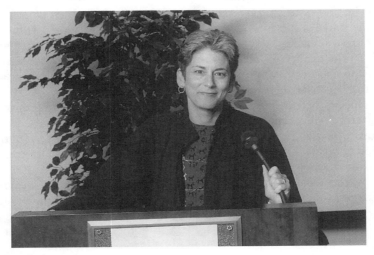

Rachel Warren

Rachel added, "We could have written the same thing about Whitehall five years ago, but thanks to your good work"—Rachel gestured by extending her arms toward the audience—"those words are less true today." Rachel paused to pick up another document. "Each of you should have a copy of the latest *Our Kids Count Coalition Community Report.*"

As the banquet guests retrieved their reports, Rachel continued, "The report tells us that, compared to five years ago, our young people are smoking less, and consuming less alcohol and other substances; alcohol-related auto crashes are down; and we are seeing better attendance in schools and fewer dropouts. Although we would like to have seen even larger differences, and we still have a long road ahead, the truth is that we are making a difference!"

The burst of applause was spontaneous. When it subsided, Rachel said: "We could not have accomplished what we have without the unselfish commitment of those of you who we honor tonight: our wonderful corps of volunteers. Now, I would like Mayor Crawford to return to the podium and, with the able assistance of Bobbie Washington, student body president of Whitehall Senior High (who, I might add, is one of our youth volunteers), make the formal presentation of awards. Mr. Mayor?"

As the awards were being presented, Rachel thought of Dick Loman and wished that he could have been there. He had moved away from the area a year before to take a new position in the Division of Adolescent and School Health at the Centers for Disease Control and Prevention in Atlanta. It had been Dick who, four years earlier, had provided the insight and leadership for bringing a much-needed focus to the coalition's planning process.

The Our Kids Count Coalition had been formed about three months after the initial workshop in March 1990. The new coalition was fueled by two sources of energy: (1) the recognition that substance abuse was a serious threat to the quality of life of Whitehall, and (2) the astute and passionate leadership of Rachel Warren, whose most obvious attribute was, paradoxically, that "just saying no" to her was not an option!

During the latter part of its first year, the coalition began preparations to submit a grant application for funding support from the Center for Substance Abuse Prevention (CSAP) in the U.S. Department of Health and Human Services. The Whitehall school board had agreed to join the coalition as the fiscal agent in the grant application.

As they undertook the background work necessary to prepare the application, some coalition members wondered if they hadn't underestimated just how complex and multidimensional the problem of substance abuse was. It was difficult for some to see just how they were going to get their arms around such a complicated issue. But Rachel had an idea!

She remembered the presentation Dick Loman had given at that initial workshop in March 1990. She got in touch with him by phone at the university. She described the goals of the Our Kids Count Coalition and explained that, in close cooperation with the Whitehall school district, they were going after a CSAP grant. Dick indicated that he was quite familiar with the CSAP grant process. Rachel explained that a small work group had been asked to take on the responsibility for preparing the grant, but as they got further into the task, it became clear that they could use help in trying to focus the application. Could he give them that help?

Dick agreed to offer assistance and suggested that before any long-term commitments were made by either him or the coalition, it would be best if he could have a preliminary meeting with the work group.

Four days later, Rachel, five members of the coalition grant application work group, and Dick Loman met at Rachel's home in Whitehall.

As he was being introduced to members of the work group, Dick was pleasantly surprised to find out that an old friend, Al Freeman, was among them. Al had been a curriculum coordinator for the state department of education and had recently taken a position as assistant principal at Whitehall Senior High.

Before the group formally gathered, Dick asked Al if Whitehall was one of the communities covered in the surveys the state department of education had been conducting since 1985 on students' knowledge, attitudes, and practices related to substance abuse. Al confirmed that Whitehall was indeed part of the sample and that the coalition had plans to make good use of the data.

Rachel ushered the group into the family room, where she had arranged the chairs and sofa in a circle to facilitate discussion. At Dick's request, Rachel began the meeting by providing a quick briefing of the coali-

1. Defined the problem: unacceptable levels of substance abuse by youth.

2. Made a clear case showing the many ways in which substance abuse compromises the quality of life of Whitehall: school dropouts and absenteeism, crime, vehicular injures, and death.

3. Received firm commitments from the local school district and multiple community agencies and organizations to support a comprehensive strategy.

4. Acquired access to data and information that would enable them to track whether changes were occurring.

FIGURE 3.1   Accomplishments of the Our Kids Count Coalition

tion's vision, its goals, its membership, and major activities to date. When she had completed her briefing, Rachel turned the floor over to Dr. Loman.

Dick thanked Rachel and then set up a flip chart he had brought with him and told the members of the work group that, from his perspective, they had a lot going for them. Then, he wrote down and commented on four of the accomplishments they had made. (See Figure 3.1.)

Dick said that all of those accomplishments would be pluses in their application, and then began to explain some of the key things grant review panels typically look for.

"They will want to know, within reasonably specific limits, what it is you intend to accomplish. Suppose you say that one of your objectives is to improve (or change in a positive direction) the attitudes and practices of kids age twelve to sixteen in Whitehall. Specifically what attitudes and what practices would you be talking about? They will also want to see some justification for selecting *those specific* attitudes and practices."

Dick paused, and then added, "Rachel told me earlier that the coalition was taking some steps to strengthen the enforcement of laws pertaining to alcohol and tobacco sales to youth. That is also a plus because when you indicate that you are proposing to implement new policies, or strengthen existing ones, you will be able to answer two of the questions the review panel will ask: Policies about what? To accomplish what end?" Members of the work group nodded, acknowledging the points Dick was making.

Then he said, "And finally, if I were a member of the panel, I would ask you this: Keeping in mind your overall goal, if you could accomplish only a portion of the things you propose, which would be the most important?"

One of the work group members, Audrey Maxfield, manager of a local Blockbuster Video store, quickly responded, "Enforcing the sales-to-minors laws. You don't use what you don't have."

Al Freeman responded to Audrey, "There's no question that we do need to enforce existing policies, but we can't stop there. We need a much better educational program for everyone in the community—not just for the kids."

Audrey defended her point of view. "He asked which would be the *most important* thing, not the *only* thing."

Dick Loman then called on his teaching experience. "You're right, Audrey. I was trying to make the point that you will have to address the matter of setting priorities, because it is highly unlikely that you will have either the time or the resources to do all of the things you want to do."

Audrey didn't hide her pleasure.

Dick continued, "On the other hand, Al has made an equally important point. To achieve your vision, you will need a strategy consisting of the right mix of activities and programs. Policy is sure to be a critical component, but what else will need to be in place if you are to realize your goal?"

Dick returned to the flip chart and said, "After my telephone conversation with Rachel earlier in the week, I took the liberty of creating an example illustrating a framework or model I have found helpful in generating information that will enable you to respond to the kind of questions I've just raised." He flipped to a new page. "I want to walk you through this diagram to give you a feel for how the model works. In doing so, I hope to share with you a way to answer the question: What causes the causes?" (See Figure 3.2.)

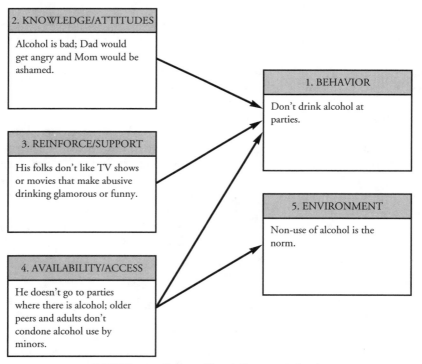

FIGURE 3.2 Factors That Influence Behavior

"In the box to your far right, numbered 1, we've stated a specific behavior of interest, in this case, youth (twelve to fourteen years of age) refusing to drink alcohol at a party. Incidentally, the process I am about to describe applies whether you are trying to understand individual behaviors, that is, one student or one patient, or collective behavior, that is, a group or community. Boxes 2, 3, 4, and 5 represent categories of different factors that have the potential of influencing that specific behavior.

"To make this simple, let's go through the process as if our target is a fourteen-year-old named Rusty. The factors in box 2 pertain to the knowledge, attitudes, and beliefs that can influence a given action.

"The data I've gathered indicate that Rusty *knows* that alcohol can impair his judgment and that it is against the law for him to drink alcohol; he also *believes* that if his dad found out that he drank, he'd be in big trouble, and if his mom found out, she'd be ashamed.

"Box 3 calls our attention to those factors that lend support for, or reinforce, a given action. Let's say that Rusty's parents express their dismay, rather than humor, over films or TV shows that portray episodes of out-of-control drinking as glamorous or funny, and that his best friends behave in ways that suggest they think drinking is stupid.

"Box 4 asks us to consider the matters of availability and accessibility. Suppose that alcohol is rarely, if ever, available at parties that Rusty goes to and that older peers and adults that he comes in contact with don't even think about making alcohol available to him or his friends.

"Box 5 contains factors that represent forces in the social environment.[1] In this instance, a variety of weekend and after-school social programs are available for youth in Rusty's age group, including athletic leagues run by police and religious groups."

With a straight face, Rachel said, "Sounds like Rusty lives in *Mister Rogers' Neighborhood!*" Everyone laughed, especially Dick. He added rhetorically, "Too good to be true, eh?"

He went to the flip chart, took out a red marking pen, drew a line through the references to Rusty's beliefs about his parents' reactions described in box 2, and wrote in "Drinking is cool." Then he pointed to box 3 and said, "Instead of what we have here, suppose I had put something like: Rusty's parents always put on dinner parties that feature a generous supply of liquor, and frequently people get intoxicated."

He then focused his attention on box 4, speaking as he wrote, "One of his best friends often drinks on weekends, getting beer from his seventeen-year-old-sister."

Rachel spoke up again. "So much for *Mister Rogers' Neighborhood!*"

"Exactly," Dick answered. "Suppose we analyzed the data we have on youth age twelve to sixteen in Whitehall, and the profile we came up with was similar to this last adjustment we made on the example with Rusty. How would this knowledge influence the way you allocate your resources? Would you direct them to programs teaching kids about the dangers of alcohol abuse? To programs teaching skills kids need to resist pressure from friends? To programs aimed at creating heightened awareness among parents—especially of how their behavior affects kids?"

The ensuing discussion was lively and productive. Dick gave several examples of how the work group could apply this diagnostic planning approach, using existing data from Whitehall, to propose some specific intervention strategies in the grant application. The group members felt as if they had a way to put the complexity into perspective—which made things seem less daunting.

The next morning, Dick called Rachel and accepted the invitation to join the work group. In the ensuing weeks, he recruited two graduate students who subsequently helped design and administer a questionnaire to collect information that would fill in a few information gaps. The work group completed the grant application on time.

Five months after the work group's meeting at Rachel's home, the Whitehall school district and the Our Kids Count Coalition were officially notified that they had received a $1.3-million grant from the Center for Substance Abuse and Prevention (CSAP).

*   *   *

After the last volunteer had been recognized, Mayor Crawford asked those gathered for one last round of appreciation. Rachel thought to herself, "Dick Loman would have liked this."

Case Analysis

In the "What Causes the Causes?" case story, we can see that the Our Kids Count Coalition evolved into a force to be reckoned with in Whitehall. Under Rachel's strong leadership, the coalition helped to heighten social consciousness about alcohol and drug abuse and, in doing so, also inspired communitywide hope for better things ahead for the young people of Whitehall. Their pursuit of the CSAP grant forced coalition members to express their hopes in more tangible terms. That process brought into sharper relief both the magnitude and complexity of the problem they were taking on—some coalition members feared that they would not be able to get a handle on a problem as complex as substance abuse.

When Dr. Loman provided the example of the diagnostic planning model, he helped members of the work group see that there was a way to get not one but several "handles" on the problem. He also helped them see the utility of probing for the factors that explain why substance abuse was a problem in Whitehall because it would give them the essential information they needed to make informed decisions about specific activities or programs.

In addition, these probes encouraged them to examine and describe the logic behind their choices—information that would be helpful not only to funding agencies, but to others as well. The remainder of this chapter provides the details one should attend to when applying the diagnostic approach described by Dr. Loman.

ASSUMPTIONS

Before practitioners get to the point where they will be applying the process that follows, we must make several assumptions.

Assumption 1: A "shared vision" has already been established for the overall program.

Assumption 2: A specific health problem has been identified and a measurable health objective has been stated.

Assumption 3: One of the program's priority tasks is to identify social/environmental conditions and behaviors that are (1) known to contribute to the health problem in question and (2) amenable to change.

Assumption 4: The program has limited time and resources.

THE TARGETS FOR CHANGE

Over the years, health promotion practitioners in school, community, clinical, and workplace settings, like Dick Loman in the case story, have found the Precede/Proceed model[2] to be a valuable tool for solving a variety of complex problems.

In the portion of the Precede/Proceed model emphasized here, we start with the task given in Assumption 3 described earlier: to identify social/environmental conditions and behaviors that are (1) known to contribute to the health problem in question and (2) amenable to change. Let's suppose that your planning group has drafted the following overall program objective:

> By the year 2000, as a result of a coordinated prevention program, reduce fatal injuries among those aged 15 to 24 caused by motor vehicle crashes in [your community] to no more than 17 per 100,000 population. (The current local rate is 33/100,000.)

Once the program objective has been established, here are the steps you would follow to get a clearer picture of the specific actions you might take to achieve that objective.

Step 1: List Risk Factors

Use your knowledge of the relevant literature and your past experience to generate a list of the potential behavioral and environmental factors known to be risk factors for motor vehicle injuries. Your list might include:

Use of seat belts
Driver's age
Air bags in car
Road conditions
Weather conditions
Driving ability
Heavy traffic
Street lighting
Illegal sale of alcohol to minors
Driving speed
Driver's gender

Speed limits
Driving under the influence of
  alcohol
Child safety seat usage
Location of crash
Time/day of week when crashes
  occur
Placement of warning signs
Laws prohibiting alcohol sales to
  minors not enforced

Step 2: Differentiate between Behavioral and Environmental Factors

Examine the list and determine which are behavioral and which are environmental. In this case, simply place a *B* for behavioral or an *E* for environmental next to each factor.

_____ Use of seat belts
_____ Driver's age
_____ Air bags in car
_____ Road conditions
_____ Weather conditions
_____ Driving ability
_____ Heavy traffic
_____ Street lighting
_____ Illegal sale of alcohol to
         minors
_____ Driving speed

_____ Driver's gender
_____ Speed limits
_____ Driving under the influence
         of alcohol
_____ Child safety seat usage
_____ Location of crash
_____ Time/day of week when
         crashes occur
_____ Placement of warning signs
_____ Laws prohibiting alcohol
         sales to minors not enforced

This may seem a tedious process. But the investment in time now can save you time later and help you avoid the frustrating and sometimes embarrassing experience of having to do it all over again!

Step 3: Shorten the List

Remember, the purpose of this process is to help you focus on those key factors that will help you achieve your program objective. The key question is: What criteria should you use to winnow the list down? By definition, practitioners are practical. They want to do things that count, things that are relevant. In this process, therefore, the ever-present question is: Which of these factors apply in this specific situation?

In addition to drawing on the experience they have gained by working with the population in question, practitioners will find rich sources of community-specific information from records kept by local police, emergency medical services, and the results of local surveys and focus-group interviews.

Suppose that local information confirms that the following six factors are relevant to the current example:

- Use of seat belts
- Driving speed
- Driving under the influence of alcohol
- Age of driver
- Driving ability
- Location of crash

To create an even more manageable list, the next step is to reexamine the factors and determine the extent to which each is *important* and *changeable.*

Step 4: Determine Importance

To determine the importance of a given factor, you need to answer two questions:

1. How prevalent is the behavior, or how frequently is the environmental factor involved?
2. Is there good evidence that the factor clearly contributes to the health problem?

Based on the information we have available to answer these questions, Figure 3.3 shows how we would rate each factor along a continuum from "More Important" to "Less Important."

Note: If your planning circumstances enable you to engage multiple experts or participants in the rating process, we would recommend creating a ten-point scale along the continuum. Ask each of the raters to identify a specific number, then add the numbers and average the ratings. Those items scoring above the midpoint of the scale can be treated as more important, and those below the midpoint, less important.

Step 5: Determine Changeability

Health promotion practitioners are charged with developing programs that will "make a difference." In most instances, that difference will be reflected

More Important   **Use of Seat Belts**   Less Important

Comment: Seat belts are used by only 27 percent of drivers involved in crashes.

More Important   **Driving Speed**   Less Important

Comment: In crashes not involving alcohol, excess speed is a factor in only 3 percent of the cases.

More Important   **Drinking and Driving**   Less Important

Comment: Forty-four percent of all motor vehicle fatalities are alcohol related; a local survey shows that 50 percent of high-school youth report that they have either driven while drinking or been with a driver who has been drinking.

More Important   **Age of Driver**   Less Important

Comment: Forty-eight percent of motor vehicle crashes involve drivers under age nineteen.

More Important   **Sales to Minors**   Less Important

Comment: A recent school-based survey of self-reported behaviors indicated that when minors try to purchase cigarettes from selected quick-stop stores or older friends, they are successful three out of four times.

More Important   **Enforcement of Laws re: Sales to Minors**   Less Important

Comment: Police records reveal that there have been no charges brought against local merchants for sale of alcoholic beverages to minors in the last three years.

FIGURE 3.3   Rating Environmental Factors by Importance

in a measurable change in a specific behavior or environmental condition. Because some behaviors and environmental factors are more or less changeable, knowledge of changeability will not only help the practitioner determine the feasibility of "making a difference," but it will also help estimate the time it will take to detect a difference.

For example, suppose there are two groups of smokers. One group consists of teenagers in Des Moines, Iowa, all of whom began smoking within the past year. The other is a group of men who live in Budapest, Hungary, all of whom are over 40 and have been smoking their entire adult lives. While the possibility of change exists for both groups, the effort and time needed to change the latter group would be far greater than that for the former!

Change is more likely to occur when a behavior is in the early developmental stages or has only recently been adopted, and when there is some expression of willingness to change on the part of the individual or group.[3] As we all know from our own life experiences, change is more difficult when the action has been long established, when it is deeply rooted in cultural practices and beliefs, when prior efforts to change have been ineffective, and when there is evidence that the individual or group in question has no interest in making a change.

Our experience is that determining the potential for change among environmental factors is less amenable to prescription, and the practitioner needs to rely on good judgment. Here are a few simple rules of thumb we have found helpful. Changeability is likely to be high if:

- There is precedence elsewhere for similar changes.

   Example: As a part of a communitywide cardiovascular disease prevention program in Wichita, Kansas, the program director wants to increase the number of restaurants that offer low-fat menu options and provide no-smoking seating areas. Similar efforts have been successful in Kansas City.

- The economic costs are not prohibitive.

   Example: Inordinately high rates of injury and death among seniors in Brooklyn, New York, have been attributed to the following: senior pedestrians have been hit by motor vehicles while trying to cross a wide street (Queens Boulevard), especially during the morning and afternoon rush hours. The majority of senior pedestrians are unable to cross Queens Boulevard in the time allotted for the green light. The light-change timing pattern has been lengthened, and speed bumps have been installed in the area.

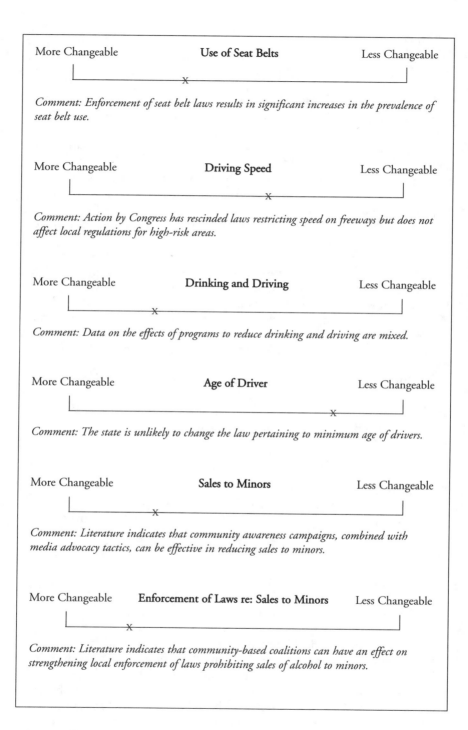

More Changeable   **Use of Seat Belts**   Less Changeable

Comment: Enforcement of seat belt laws results in significant increases in the prevalence of seat belt use.

More Changeable   **Driving Speed**   Less Changeable

Comment: Action by Congress has rescinded laws restricting speed on freeways but does not affect local regulations for high-risk areas.

More Changeable   **Drinking and Driving**   Less Changeable

Comment: Data on the effects of programs to reduce drinking and driving are mixed.

More Changeable   **Age of Driver**   Less Changeable

Comment: The state is unlikely to change the law pertaining to minimum age of drivers.

More Changeable   **Sales to Minors**   Less Changeable

Comment: Literature indicates that community awareness campaigns, combined with media advocacy tactics, can be effective in reducing sales to minors.

More Changeable   **Enforcement of Laws re: Sales to Minors**   Less Changeable

Comment: Literature indicates that community-based coalitions can have an effect on strengthening local enforcement of laws prohibiting sales of alcohol to minors.

FIGURE 3.4   Rating Environmental Factors by Changeability

More Important   Less Important

More Changeable	• Drinking and Driving • Sales to Minors • Enforcement of Laws • Use of Seat Belts Quadrant 1	• Driving Speed Quadrant 3
Less Changeable	• Age of Driver Quadrant 2	 Quadrant 4

FIGURE 3.5 Importance and Changeability Matrix

- The proposed change is supported by public demand.

    Example: Most observers agree that a significant part of the success of the well-documented North Karelia Project can be attributed to its ability to educate the public and thereby create a public demand for the food industry to increase its production of skim milk and low-fat dairy products.

    Again, based on the information we have, Figure 3.4 shows how we would position each factor along a continuum from "More Changeable" to "Less changeable."

Step 6: Create a Matrix

Information from your importance and changeability analyses will enable you to create a single "picture" in the form of a simple 2-by-2 matrix like the one shown in Figure 3.5. Using the same ratings applied on each continuum, the matrix reveals how the various factors "cluster" in terms of importance and changeability.

The factors that end up in quadrant 1 are those that are both important and changeable. As such, they are likely to be prime candidates for focus in your health promotion program.

In this example the age of the driver is deemed important but less changeable, and therefore is placed in quadrant 2. The rating of high importance was made based on the fact that nearly half of all crashes involved drivers under the age of nineteen.

Although one cannot literally change age, figuratively it is changeable in the sense that the minimum age for obtaining a driver's license might be changed from the current sixteen years of age to eighteen. Eliminating the rule permitting earlier licensing if a teenager takes a driver education course is one way of changing the average age of drivers.

In most instances, factors deemed highly important but less changeable are good targets for an innovative intervention if accompanied by careful evaluation. Evidence from such evaluations that a new approach can change a given factor could then be used to argue for greater changeability and wider application of that approach.

For example, suppose you are planning a program designed to reduce sexual promiscuity and unprotected sex among a culturally diverse population of teens. You read an article by Dan Romer and his colleagues,[6] which describes a strategy wherein a group of parents in an African-American neighborhood shared the responsibility for monitoring the actions of children and youth within their "friendship network." The effect of this approach was a marked reduction in sexual activity. You acknowledge the importance of parental supervision, and this approach makes good intuitive sense to you.

Nevertheless, you can't be certain how feasible it would be to implement such a strategy in the population you are serving. In that case, you would likely list "Parental Monitoring" in quadrant 2 and make certain that the appropriate steps are taken to assess the extent to which it (1) was properly implemented and (2) had an effect on your program objective.

Step 7: Set Objectives

The potential effectiveness of a health promotion program can be jeopardized when the objectives are stated in vague language and thus are difficult to measure. Given the assumption that practitioners have limited time and resources, vagueness is not a prudent option. When behavior change is deemed important and possible, care must be taken to state objectives with care and precision.[4] Such objectives should answer these questions:

Who? (the people expected to change)

What? (the action or change to be achieved)

How much? (the extent of the condition to be achieved)

When? (the time in which the change is expected to occur)

Here are sample objectives for two of the factors that appear in quadrant 1:

- **Drinking and Driving** (Behavioral Factor). By September of the year 2000, reduce by 50 percent the number of youth age sixteen to eighteen who report that they drink and drive.
- **Sales to Minors** (Environmental Factor). By June of 1998, local government authorities will implement and actively support a policy calling for full enforcement of laws prohibiting sales of alcohol to minors.

IDENTIFYING THE CAUSES

Once the priority behavioral and environmental objectives have been determined, planners need to answer this question: What factors seem to be contributing to the behavioral and environmental conditions that we seek to influence? Once those candidates have been identified, many of the steps used to determine importance and changeability will be repeated.

We make the assumption that all behavioral and environmental targets are shaped by a variety of factors and conditions, some of which are likely to have more influence on outcomes than others. This variety is a reflection of the complexity that is inherent when dealing with any human/social problem. Accountable health promotion practitioners cannot deny that complexity; they can only work within it. A portion of the Precede/Proceed model includes a graphic framework to help practitioners manage that complexity. Figure 3.6 provides an illustration of that framework.

Predisposing factors help practitioners to cluster and examine how *cognitive capacities* (what we know) and *affective characteristics* (how we feel and what we believe in) might influence a specific pattern of behavior. For example, (1) the absence of knowledge, (2) the belief that one has no control over what happens to him or her, and (3) feelings of low self-confidence regarding changing the behavior in question are modifiable characteristics that can put an individual or group at unnecessary risk.

We have often heard the comment that when it comes right down to it, knowledge plays a very small role in influencing behavior. An example of this attitude might be: "Teen smokers will not give up their habit because you tell them they will be 20 times more likely to die from lung cancer than those who don't smoke by the time they reach the age of 55." While the example is a good one, it does not merit the generalization that knowledge is comparatively unimportant.

Suppose you have been assigned to work in a region of Nigeria where malaria is the leading cause of death and disability. It has been determined that pockets of standing water, which could be readily cleaned up, are the primary breeding grounds for mosquitoes. To what extent would a cultural-

```
┌─────────────────────────────────────────┐
│           Predisposing Factors           │
│   (Factors that provide a rationale or   │
│   motivate action)                       │
│                                          │
│              • Knowledge                 │
│              • Attitudes                 │
│              • Beliefs                   │
│              • Values                    │
│              • Perception                │
│                                          │
└─────────────────────────────────────────┘
```

```
┌─────────────────────────────────────────┐   ┌─────────────────────────────────────────┐
│           Reinforcing Factors            │   │          Behavioral Objective            │
│   (Interpersonal [human] actions that    │   │                                          │
│   reward or support a given behavior)    │   │   • Measurable statement of an action    │
│                                          │   │     to be taken by a given point in time │
│       • Attitudes and actions of         │   │                                          │
│         teachers, peers, staff, and      │   │                                          │
│         parents                          │   │                                          │
│                                          │   │                                          │
└─────────────────────────────────────────┘   └─────────────────────────────────────────┘
```

```
┌─────────────────────────────────────────┐   ┌─────────────────────────────────────────┐
│            Enabling Factors              │   │         Environmental Objective          │
│   (Factors that enable an action to be   │   │                                          │
│   taken)                                 │   │   • Measurable statement of a social     │
│                                          │   │     or environmental condition to be     │
│       • Availability and accessibility   │   │     attained by a given point in time    │
│         of educational resources and     │   │                                          │
│         supportive policies and systems  │   │                                          │
│                                          │   │                                          │
└─────────────────────────────────────────┘   └─────────────────────────────────────────┘
```

FIGURE 3.6   Predisposing, Reinforcing, and Enabling Factors

ly sensitive understanding of this knowledge be of importance to the villagers and their leaders?

The point we wish to make is this: The value of an analytic process like the one we are using here is that it asks practitioners to assess the reality and circumstances under which they are working. Depending upon that reality, knowledge may or may not be a critical factor; such a decision can be made only after thoughtful review.

Some practitioners refer to **reinforcing factors** in terms of the notion of feedback. That fits! Reinforcement is feedback with effect; feedback rewards the action taken. The attitudes and climate of support one gets (or doesn't get) can have a very strong influence on behavior. Thus, it should be a priority to determine the role that parents, family members, co-workers, peers, best friends, health care providers, supervisors, and other people play in supporting or discouraging a given behavior. Because exposure to the media also falls into this category, similar consideration should be given to print, film, and electronic media, including the Internet.

Those conditions of the environment that facilitate actions by individuals, groups, or organizations are called **enabling factors.** The extent to which services, facilities, programs, or program elements are available, accessible, and/or affordable are good examples of this factor. Negative examples include:

- encouraging low-income women over age 50 to seek mammograms while failing to take into account that mammograms are (1) available only during hours that the women are working and (2) are unaffordable for them.
- promoting a tobacco-use prevention and control program for youth without addressing the reality that tobacco vending machines are ubiquitous.

Also included under this category are the specific skills one needs to perform a given behavior. Skills and reinforcement can be interdependent. To illustrate this point, consider the following example. Several years ago, a group of physicians wanted us to help teach senior citizens with hypertension how to take each other's blood pressure. The physicians hoped that teaching the seniors those skills would result in a decrease in the number of unnecessary office visits.

We decided to do a small pilot study. The seniors were randomly assigned to either an intervention group or a control group. Intervention subjects were taught how to use the sphygmomanometer and stethoscope on one another and record the readings. We had experienced previous success using similar methods with junior-high students.

As a part of the formative aspect of our evaluation plan, we had scheduled one site visit a week. During the first visit, the signs of impending disaster were already apparent. Although most of the participants reported that they felt pleased and empowered with their new ability, the remainder were frustrated and indicated that the program made them downright angry—it reminded them of their shortcomings. The causes were multiple: their arthritis prohibited them from squeezing the bulb on the sphygmomanometer, or their vision was too impaired to read the measurement, or they couldn't hear the stethoscope. Feedback was immediate. But it was discouraging rather than rewarding, so it did not maintain the behavior.

Our failure to do a thorough job of assessing enabling factors (which in this instance were mostly physical) led to negative rather than positive feedback and a well-intended but flawed intervention program. More important, it was a program that, left unchecked, could do harm!

GENERATING PREDISPOSING, REINFORCING, AND ENABLING FACTORS

To get a sense of how to apply this level of analysis, let's return to one of the objectives stated earlier:

> By September of the year 2000, reduce by 50 percent the number of youth age sixteen to eighteen who report that they drink and drive.

Step 1. Generate a list of factors that may affect or explain why young people in your community choose to drink and drive.

- Teens do not perceive themselves to be at risk—"It won't happen to me"
- Police know the likely days/times of crashes, but don't patrol
- The media glamorize beer
- The mayor thinks teen drinking and driving is an important issue
- Eighty-five percent of teens report they know the dangers of drinking and driving
- Many parents believe that taking drugs, not drinking alcohol, is the problem
- Alcohol at teen parties is a tradition
- Laws prohibiting sales to minors are not enforced

Step 2. Classify them into predisposing, reinforcing, and enabling factors. Figure 3.7 presents an illustration of how the factors generated in Step 1 fall into the three categories.

The remainder of the process follows exactly the same steps you followed in the previous exercise.

Step 3. Using the same criteria you applied earlier, determine the importance of each factor.

Step 4. Repeat the same process to determine the changeability of each factor.

Step 5. Create a matrix to help you visualize the factors that have the highest importance and changeability ratings.

Step 6. For each factor that you chose to focus upon, state a measurable objective that incorporates the essential elements of this question: *Who* will do *how much* of *what* by *when*?

Predisposing Factors
• Teens do not perceive themselves to be at risk—"It won't happen to me" • Merchants do not think they will be prosecuted for selling alcohol to minors

Reinforcing Factors	Behavioral Objective
• Many parents believe that drugs, not alcohol, are the problem • Laws prohibiting sales to minors are not enforced • The media glamorize beer • The mayor thinks teen drinking and driving is an important issue	• By September of the year 2000, reduce by 50 percent the number of youth aged sixteen to eighteen who report that they drink and drive

Enabling Factors	Environmental Objective
• Alcohol at teen parties is a tradition • It is easy to buy alcohol	• Reduce sales of alcohol to minors by 50 percent by 1999

FIGURE 3.7   Factors That Influence Teen Drinking and Driving

G'DAY: AUSTRALIA'S DIAGNOSTIC APPROACH

This diagnostic process has been used in literally hundreds of applications around the world. In 1996, we had the opportunity to visit a project underway in Western Australia, where researchers at Curtin University and local school officials in Perth were working on an intervention to reduce child pedestrian injuries, the leading cause of death and severe injury in children in Western Australia. In the office where the central planning for the project was carried out, a modified version of this diagnostic approach was posted on the wall as a large working flow chart; the Australian group used this flow chart to keep members of the team focused on their specific tasks within the context of the overall program strategy. With permission from the Australian researchers and practitioners[5] directing that project, we have recreated that chart as Tables 3.1 and 3.2. As you scan the tables, note how the specific objectives have been included along the way.

TABLE 3.1 Preventing Pedestrian Injuries among Five-to-Nine-Year-Olds

Behavioral Factors	Contributing Factors	Intervention Strategy Selection
RF *Children crossing roads* O Reduce % of children crossing at busy roads O Increase % of children crossing at safer sites	*Belief of children—low perception of risk re crossing busy roads* SO Develop beliefs of children *Lack of environmental supports* SO ID safer sites *Knowledge of children re road-crossing behaviors (RCB)* SO Enhance knowledge of children	StO School education: 1. develop beliefs of children re risk of crossing busy roads 2. ID alternative "safer" routes, map routes, etc. 3. ID "safer" crossing sites StO Parent education on child pedestrian safety StO Environmental: improve signs, paint curbs, increase number of crossing attendants
RF *Inappropriate crossing behavior by 5 to 9-year-olds* O Improve children's road-crossing behaviors O Improve children's "search" behaviors	*Beliefs of children—perception of invulnerability, etc.* SO Develop beliefs of children *Road-crossing skills of children* SO Enhance road-crossing skills of children *Inadequate family modeling of RCB* SO Improve family modeling	StO Create action/experience/modeling school pedestrian safety education program StO Provide teacher training and follow-up support to ensure implementation of the school pedestrian safety education program StO Create a parent pedestrian safety education program
RF *Children not getting help to cross roads* O Increase % of children getting help to cross roads	*Inadequate school-based road safety education* SO Implement quality road safety education *Parents' perceptions of children's abilities to cross roads safely* SO Change parents' perceptions	StO Create action/experience/modeling school pedestrian safety education program

Lack of supervision of children by parents
SO Improve appropriate supervision by parents

Social skills (decision making, assertive communication) demonstrated by children when asking people to help them cross roads
SO Enhance social skills of children

Parent perceptions of child's abilities to cross roads safely
SO Change parents' perceptions

StO Create a parent pedestrian safety education program

RF *Parents not supervising children at crossings*
O Increase % of parents supervising children at road crossings

RF *Parents not teaching appropriate road-crossing procedures*
O Increase % of parents teaching children appropriate road-crossing procedures

RF *Parents not modeling appropriate road-crossing behaviors*
O Increase % of parents modeling appropriate road-crossing behaviors

Legend:
RF = risk factor
O = objective
SO = sub-objective
StO = strategic objective

TABLE 3.2 Environmental Factors—Volume and Speed of Traffic, Road Design, Roadside Obstacles

	Environmental Factors	Contributing Factors	Intervention Strategy
RF	*High volume of traffic on residential streets*	*Posted residential speed limits too high*	StO *Inform council and state government
O	Reduce residential traffic volume (% reduction in traffic volume, construction of speed control measures)	SO Reduce posted residential speed limit	StO Inform council to redesign and replan roads
		Road design in residential areas encourages speeding and high traffic volume	StO Inform police to enforce residential speed limits
		SO Change road design	StO Develop community education campaign/ programs
		SO Council to redesign and replan	
RF	*Speed of vehicles too fast on residential streets*	*Drivers exceeding posted speed limit—Lack of enforcement*	
O	Reduce speed of vehicles (% reduction in average speed)	SO Police to enforce residential speed limits	
		Beliefs of drivers—low perception of being caught by police or causing injury	
		SO Change beliefs of drivers	
		Knowledge of drivers re children's road-crossing capabilities, etc.	
		SO Change knowledge of drivers	
		Lack of community road safety education	
		SO Develop community road safety program	

RF *Road design exposes children to busy roads*

O Redesign road hierarchy to reduce traffic volume

(% reduction in traffic volume—changes in road hierarchy)

RF *Road hierarchy design encourages speeding in residential areas*

O Redesign road hierarchy to reduce traffic speed on local streets

(% reduction in traffic speed—changes in road hierarchy)

Road hierarchy designs need coordination

    SO State government to modify road hierarchy plan

    SO Council to redesign and replan roads

Road design in residential areas encourages speeding and traffic volume

    SO Change road design

        StO Inform state government re road hierarchy plan

        StO Inform council to redesign and replan

RF *Roadside obstacles obscuring children*

O Reduce obscuring obstacles

O Relocate/redesign structures (posts/booths)

O Restrict parking/alternative parking

Knowledge or perception of council staff and community about roadside obstacles

    SO Change knowledge/perception of council staff and community

        StO Develop community education campaign/ programs

        StO Inform staff/authorities, etc.

Legend:

RF = risk factor

O = objective

SO = sub-objective

StO = strategic objective

*Inform through advocacy and information campaigns

SUMMARY

How often we have heard the story of caring practitioners—with virtually no resources to obtain baseline data or evaluation—who use their experience and knowledge of local circumstances to create innovative programs, after which local observers express the strong sentiment and belief that the program "worked" or "made a difference." However, when the time inevitably comes to demonstrate the effect of such programs, the practitioner discovers that sentiment is no match for documented evidence.

We suspect that in many of these instances, there probably are genuine effects, most of which unfortunately go undetected. If practitioners adopt the analytic approach suggested in this chapter, they will automatically build in the essential ingredients required to make their program efforts evaluable. By identifying priority problems and the behavioral and environmental risks associated with those problems, by framing measurable objectives and creating specific tactics to achieve those objectives, you put into place the markers for evaluation. By taking this kind of accountable approach, practitioners will find, just as Rachel Warren discovered, that recruiting evaluation partners—including economic support—is much easier.

ENDNOTES

1. In this context, we refer to "environmental factors" primarily as the social conditions that can have a direct or indirect influence on either a health behavior or a specific health problem. For example, organizational or social policies (laws pertaining to the sale of tobacco to youth, speed limits, indoor clear air acts, health insurance regulations, standards for screening and immunization, etc.). In some instances, the physical environment may be especially relevant as in the case of poor road conditions, insufficient lighting in a building, standing water that breeds mosquitoes, lead paint and dust.

2. Green LW, Kreuter MW. *Health Promotion Planning: An Educational and Environmental Approach.* Menlo Park, CA: Mayfield Publishing; 1990. To date, there have been over 500 published accounts of the model.

3. The basic assumption underlying stages-of-change theory is that behavior change can be best understood as a process of steps or stages of transition from resistance to taking a given action to taking and repeating that action. For a good review of the theory, we suggest: Prochaska JO, DiClemente CC, Norcross JC. In search of how people change: applications to addictive behaviors. *Am Psychologist.* 1992; 47:1102–1114.

4. The primary difference between stating objectives for behaviors and for environmental factors is that the *who* question is usually not included in stating the environmental objective.

5. We are grateful to Donna Cross, Peter Howatt, Steve Jones, Mark Stevenson, and Margaret Hall and their colleagues at the Centre of Health Promotion Research at Curtin University in Perth, Australia, for allowing us to use the

adaptation of the Precede/Proceed model they have employed to guide their research and development of the Child Pedestrian Injury Prevention Project in Western Australia.

6. Romer D, Black M, Ricardo I, Feigelman S, Daljee L, Galbraith J, et al. Social influences of youth at risk for HIV exposure. *Am J Public Health.* 1994;84(6): 977–985.

CHAPTER 4

Promoting Social Capital

Case Story
THE COURT OF PUBLIC OPINION

It was nearly 6:30 P.M. and almost everyone had gone home an hour before. Ray Wycoff sat quietly at his desk, mindlessly elaborating on a series of circles he had sketched on the back of an envelope. It had been a long and frustrating day in what seemed to be a year's worth of long and frustrating days. The knock at the door startled him.

"Yes?"

The door opened slowly, leaving an opening large enough to frame the smiling face of Adam Solomon. "Planning to sleep over?"

Ray smiled. "What are you doing here?" In addition to being a neighbor and good friend, Adam Solomon was the managing editor for Hillsdale's daily paper, the *Sentinel-Dispatch,* and his office was located a block and a half from the Hillsdale Health Department.

"Hey, I'm a taxpayer and this is public property isn't it?" Adam laughed. "I saw the light on in your office, and I need a ride home—the garage didn't have the parts in stock to fix my car so they had to keep it overnight."

Ray had always marveled at Adam, who at 34 was probably one of the youngest managing editors in the country. Although his work inevitably put him at the hub of political controversy, he was always on an even keel; his trademark was his irresistible sense of humor. Ray gestured toward the door as he got up. "Your taxi is waiting, sir!"

During the ride home, Ray was quiet and self-absorbed. "You look a little down," Adam observed. "What's up? Or down, as the case may be?"

Ray thought for a moment and then said, "Bottom line: I have come to the realization that I'm having a heck of a hard time doing the job I was hired to do and want to do!"

"You can't be serious!" Adam said, studying the expression on his friend's face. Then he added, "You are serious. What's going on?"

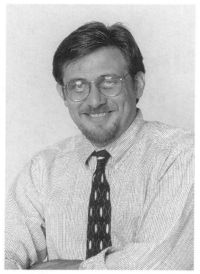

Ray Wycoff

Ray didn't answer. He just pursed his lips and slowly shook his head from side to side.

Adam knew that Ray's wife, Jeanne, had taken their two children to her mother's home in upstate New York. As Ray turned into Adam's driveway, Adam said, "Since Jeanne is out of town, why don't you have dinner with Susan and me?"

"Ray shook his head. "Thanks anyway, I've got some work to do."

"It's no trouble, and work or no work, you've got to eat. Besides, I'd like to hear more about not being able to do your job. How about a beer?"

"Sure, a beer sounds good. Why not?"

There was a note on the kitchen table:

Adam:

Gone to office to finish up a document for a closing we have tomorrow A.M. Back about 8:30. Will bring pizza.

Love you, Susan

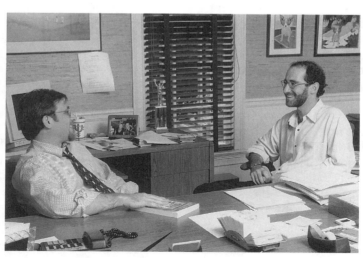

Ray Wycoff and Adam Solomon

Adam held the note up and announced: "Susan's at the real estate office. She'll be home in an hour or so with some mouth-watering cuisine from Italy. Perfect!"

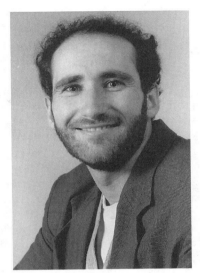

Adam Solomon

The two men sat in canvas garden chairs on the back porch. Adam raised his beer bottle to gesture a toast and Ray followed suit. "To solving problems!" Ray smiled.

Refreshed by drink, Adam declared, "OK, let's have at it. What's the problem?"

Ray paused a moment and then responded with a question of his own: "What would you do if you had information about a conspiracy in state government, information that you were able to determine was valid, and you were about to print it, only to have the governor inform you that you couldn't run it in the *Sentinel-Dispatch* or give it to anyone else?"

"Well, I'd remind Governor Baker that we have this little document called the Constitution, which has these amendments called the Bill of Rights. Then I'd direct his attention to *numero uno,* and then, after those courtesies, I'd print it!"

"Why would you print it?"

"You know very well why: In a democratic society, people have a right to know what is going on and, at the same time, the press has a moral obligation to inform the public of what's going on—hence the expression *free press.* But I don't have to tell you that. What does all of this have to do with a director of public health who thinks he and his co-workers can't do their jobs?"

"Well, we are coming to the point where my colleagues and I are being told that we can't, metaphorically speaking, print the public health truth."

"Tell me more."

"We are being told in no uncertain terms that if we act on what we know to be the truth, what science tells us is the truth, our funds will be cut and our jobs will be at risk. We're stymied and we have no health 'bill of rights' to back us up."

Adam smiled. "That's a bit dramatic, isn't it? Besides, you folks are doing a lot—how about that Kids First campaign our paper helped you promote two years ago? Within a year, immunization coverage in Hillsdale reached its highest rate in history. Incidentally, I figure you guys couldn't buy the kind of coverage we gave you."

"OK, point well taken, but there are still very important areas where we are simply being told: *hands off.*"

"By the governor?"

"Of course not."

"By whom, then?"

"Policymakers who themselves have been pressured by special-interest groups because those interest groups perceive our initiatives to be at odds with their special interests!"

With a hint of sarcasm, Adam interrupted. "We wouldn't be referring to the tobacco industry, the NRA, or the housing folks opposed to lead clean-up, would we?"

"Yes, we would. The pressure is all over the place. Last month I was at a meeting of epidemiologists from the military. They told me that a proposal to prohibit cigarette sales on military bases had been put forth and approved by the Department of Defense. They discovered later that the proposal had been tabled after members of Congress from certain tobacco-growing states had threatened to cut appropriations for base PXs. That's the kind of thing I'm talking about."

Adam grinned and stretched his arms upward, "Ah, sweet politics."

"It's not very funny to me, my friend."

Adam's smile disappeared. "From where I sit, public health is, by definition, political. And until you and your colleagues acknowledge that reality, and figure out how to operate within it, I suspect you'll probably continue to feel the way you do."

"Acknowledge it? Hell, we live it! Besides, there are very specific laws that prohibit public employees from lobbying for their causes."

"*Au contraire,* Ray. The problem is that you *don't* live it, you grudgingly *tolerate* it! I hear you saying that you are a recipient of the effects of being in a political arena; you're a victim. Frankly, I think that people outside your circle of colleagues will find that sounding a little like whining. If you want to avoid political victimization and the feeling of paralysis that inevitably accompanies it, then you have to become a player."

Ray stood up and strolled out onto the lawn behind the porch.

Adam got up and followed him, fearing that he had gone too far and offended his friend. "Hey, I didn't mean to come on so strong."

"Actually, that's not what I was thinking at all. I suppose I do sound a bit whiny. Keep going."

"What I mean by *becoming a player* is to think and act proactively. So instead of hoping that someone or some group won't raise a red flag when you put forth a new or potentially controversial program, anticipate and plan for such a reaction. To do that, and again this is admittedly my communications bias, you need to develop an ongoing strategy to let people know who you are, what you do, and why what you do is of value to the folks in this community."

When Ray responded, he couldn't mask his sarcasm. "In other words, advertise!"

"Sounds as if you equate advertising with prostitution!"

Ray was silent.

Adam continued. "Tell me, do you really think the intent of advertising is that much different from the intent of what you call education and promotion?"

Ray got the point. "We're health people; we're not trained to go around telling people how good we are—"

Adam interrupted. "Well, maybe you should be!"

"Look, we're so damn busy just keeping our heads above water, we don't have time to toot our own horns, even if we were of a mind to do so."

Adam paused and said, "I think you've got to *make* time. We're talking priorities here, and that 'tooting your own horn' remark reflects an attitude that may be a big part of the problem."

"How so?" Ray asked.

"Would you agree that people in any community will speak out and support the institutions they value if those same institutions were somehow threatened?"

Ray nodded in agreement. Sounding like a trial lawyer, Adam continued. "Would you also agree that, currently, the public's general understanding of and appreciation for public health services is probably minimal?"

"Probably."

Adam looked at Ray and slowly enunciated, "That's . . . the . . . point!" pointing at his friend to emphasize each word. "How can you expect the people of Hillsdale to be supportive, especially in the face of political pressure and opposition from special interests, if they don't know what you do and why it is in their best interest for you to have their support to keep doing it? Incidentally, you need to understand that our paper does not, *de facto,* have a responsibility to promote public health! If you created a strategy to bring the merits of public health to the court of public opinion, two things would happen and they are both good."

"I assume that you will elaborate on those two things?" Ray asked knowingly.

"Of course. First, you would educate the community and probably make 'friends' for public health that you wouldn't make otherwise. And second, that constant flow of information would serve to minimize the sensational effect that adversarial special-interest groups rely on."

Adam's reference to making 'friends' triggered memories for Ray.

"The mention of 'friends' of public health reminds me of an experience I had in my first year as health officer for the Greene County Health Department in Illinois."

"I have a nose for stories and I sense one coming on."

"Can you tolerate it?" Ray asked.

"Only if it has a good title."

Ray thought for a moment and then said, "Let's call it 'Making Friends the Hard Way'!" He described how his health department had received a planning grant to put together an injury-prevention project proposal for a target area in the county. He explained that the proposal made good use of existing county-based data and highlighted the fact that his health department had established strong collaboration with key county agencies, including the department of roads and transportation, emergency medical services, and the county sheriff's department. Ray had been adamant about his desire to secure the cooperation of other agencies. The planning team developed an impressive proposal that focused on reducing auto-related injuries among teenagers.

Ray explained that the week the proposal was due for submission to the state capital, he was asked to give a luncheon address at the Greene County Rotary Club meeting. He recalled how he had prepared his remarks to make the point that contemporary health problems are complex and not likely to be resolved without extensive cooperation among many sectors of the community.

To illustrate his point, Ray used the proposed injury-prevention program as a concrete illustration of action underway. With great enthusiasm, he described key elements of the program and showed a county map, highlighting the high-priority target areas.

The discussion period following his presentation was a disaster. It began when a coach from the high school indicated that he strongly favored an injury-prevention program, but that this was the first he had heard about it; he asked if it was too late to involve the school system, implying that the school district had been left out. Ray knew that there had been a school representative on the planning committee, but she had left the area at the end of the school year to take a new position in another part of the state. Most of the planning had taken place in the summer and no replacement had been found.

"Once the coach had spoken, I felt like I was the bait for a shark's feeding frenzy."

Adam was now fully engaged. "What happened?"

Ray described how Reverend Carver, the next speaker, stood up and politely but firmly questioned the department's priorities. The reverend observed that the main target area for the program was adjacent to low-income neighborhoods with serious housing, employment, and basic health needs.

Ray stretched his right arm up about a foot over his own head, and looked at Adam. "Reverend Carver is an imposing figure—a big man with a soft voice. As I recall, he said something like: 'Once again we see another example of the government deciding what the people want and need. The residents of the West End, which my church serves, are poor, and like all poor people, they bear a greater burden of illness than the rest of the community. Wouldn't it make more sense to spend your resources on the real causes of poor health—things like inferior housing and no jobs?'"

Ray explained how futile it was to try to explain that he understood the reverend's point, but that the money for the injury-prevention program was earmarked for injury prevention and could not be used for matters like housing and unemployment.

"The reverend politely heard my response, then rhetorically asked: 'Why not?' and sat down. I had no retort."

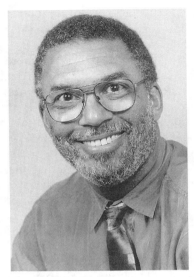

Reverend Carver

"And then you made friends?" Adam asked.

"No, then the floodgates opened. Others expressed their concerns. The most notable was the director of Mothers Against Drunk Driving, who indicated that while she was pleased to hear that the health department was getting involved with this important problem, she was disappointed to have to hear about it in a public meeting at a point when the program was apparently a *fait accompli*. She expressed disappointment at being ignored in the planning effort, even though MADD had been successful in bringing stiffer law enforcement and penalties for driving under the influence of alcohol."

Ray paused to sip his beer. "I was stunned. If I had been talking about the merits of sex education as a means to prevent the spread of HIV/AIDS, or even water fluoridation, I would have anticipated some flack, but injury prevention?"

Adam's nod reflected his understanding. "There's a real difference between *doing something with a group* and *getting it done to you*. Where does the making friends part come in?"

"Well," Ray said, "the next day, I made an appointment to meet with Reverend Carver out in the West End. I was motivated partly because I wanted to mend the fences, but also to learn what went wrong. What I discovered wasn't earthshaking or complicated...." He paused in midsentence and said, "Funny, isn't it?"

"What's that?" Adam asked.

"When you cut through all the theories and words, good communication comes down to having respect for people's views. It means taking the time to be respectful."

By urging him to be more aggressive about taking the story of public health to the public, Adam had helped Ray see the connection between increasing community awareness about the value of public health and grassroots participation. Adam also made Ray realize that community participation in public health wouldn't occur unless he made it a priority to meet with people and listen to them.

Adam thought for a moment and then spoke. "You know, most leaders and managers are struggling with change just like you are. For most of us, the social context in which we do our work has changed, but we haven't. It's as if we're experienced players in a game where the rules have been radically changed!"

"And those changes for me are political?"

"It seems that way to me. But when you say *political,* it's as if you're saying *corrupt;* and earlier you said that as a public employee, you couldn't lobby. That tells me that you believe that you have to lobby or buy favors to be a player in the political arena."

"A lot of people feel that way."

"Wait here a minute!" Adam moved briskly into the house. A few moments later he returned, carrying a huge dictionary and a thin red paperback. He put the small book down and began to flip through the pages of the dictionary. "Remember, I'm a newspaper guy and words are my business, and *political* is a big word. Ah, here we are."

Adam handed Ray the dictionary and pointed to a spot on the page. "Scan these definitions, starting with the word *politic,* through to *politicize.*"

Ray read to himself and then said, "Here it is. 'Crafty,' 'unscrupulous'. . . here's a good one, listen to this: '. . . scheming, opportunism, etc., as opposed to a *statesman,* which suggests able, far-seeing, principled conduct.' I love the 'etc.' part! I rest my case." Ray felt like a poker player who had just successfully drawn to an inside straight.

Adam grinned. "By resting your case, my friend, you have helped me make mine! One of the curious things about the words *politics, political,* and *politician* is that they have two sides: a negative side, which you chose to highlight, and a positive side, which you chose to ignore. Allow me." Adam took the dictionary from Ray's hands, studied the page for a moment, and said, "For example, you didn't mention such things as 'having practical wisdom,' 'prudent,' 'diplomatic,' 'concerned with government'—or how about this under *political liberty*: 'the right to participate in determining the form, choosing the officials, making the laws, and carrying on the function of one's government'?"

Adam handed the dictionary to Ray and picked up the paperback. "There's a phrase in here I have always liked. Ah, here it is. He cleared his throat to dramatize his reading. " . . .the term *political* is not inherently negative; it comes from the Greek notion of *polis* and refers to a place where governance was achieved through dialogue and advocacy, and it is balanced by study and inquiry."[1] He looked at Ray, "A bit idealistic, perhaps, but nice—don't you think?"

Ray thought to himself, *A full house beats a straight!* "Yes, very nice. Point well taken."

Adam went on, "For centuries, playwrights and novelists have dramatized humanity's struggle with the forces of good and evil, and the political arena has been one of the prime settings for playing out that struggle. Rather than being inherently good or bad, politics is just real. One can be a greedy and corrupt player, or one who plays with principles and dignity. For you public health folks, the choice isn't whether to play, but how you're going to balance the struggle in favor of integrity."

At that moment, Susan pulled back the sliding door to the back porch and announced, "Anyone for a little pizza with fresh eggplant, mushrooms, tomatoes, black olives, and pepperoni?"

Case Analysis

We wonder how many community health workers, with the heartfelt intentions of a Don Quixote, have had their dreams dashed by the churning blades of political windmills? The "Court of Public Opinion" case story calls our attention to the reality that social and political forces do indeed influence the ability of practitioners to plan and deliver effective community health promotion programs. In Ray Wycoff's conversation with his friend Adam Solomon, we are reminded (1) that public health practice is inseparably tied to the political workings of the community it seeks to serve; (2) that it is unreasonable to think that effective public health practice can be implemented and sustained if it is invisible to the general public and community decision makers; and, (3) that failure to seek and respect the counsel of citizens reflects a flaw in both the ethics and the application of public health programs.

The remainder of this chapter is divided into three sections offering ideas and actions that will help health promotion practitioners work more effectively within the political realities of the communities they serve. In the first section, "Making the Case", we outline a strategic approach to increase awareness about the purpose and value of public health. This section also describes tactics for reaching various audiences.

The second section, "Participation", begins with a review of the scientific and ethical rationale for actively seeking citizen participation and concludes with some practical approaches for securing that participation.

In the third section, titled "Social Capital," we make the case that an understanding of the theory of social capital will benefit practitioners as they try to work with and through communities.

MAKING THE CASE

From Geoffrey Rose's insightful book, *The Strategy of Preventive Medicine,* we find this wisdom:

> Political decisions are for the politicians. Their agenda is complex, and mostly hidden from public scrutiny. This is unfortunate, because often the public would give higher priority to health than those who formulate political policies. Anything that stimulates more public information and debate on health issues is good, not just because it may lead to healthier choices, but also because it earns a high place for health issues on the political agenda. In the long run, this is probably the most important achievement of health education.[2]

Professor Rose would have been a good reference to reinforce Adam Solomon's "prompting" of Ray Wycoff. Rose's insight also was empirically confirmed in a 1994 study conducted by Macro International and funded by the CDC.[3] A part of the study sought to ascertain the extent to which the American public understands the goals, purpose, and value of public health. Findings from the study suggested that the average citizen has little or no understanding of either the scope or the significance of public health. For example, when citizens were asked, "What comes to mind when I mention public health?" typical responses included:

- "restaurant inspections"
- "free immunizations"
- "doctors for the poor"
- "the ugly pink building downtown"

More specifically, the study identified several misperceptions and attitudes that, if unaddressed, would tend to undermine efforts to create support for public health. These included:

- limited awareness of public health's scope and significance
- strong and exclusive association of public health and health departments as one and the same, delivering services for the poor
- misplaced confidence that public health functions can be and will be performed by others (the National Guard, in one example!)
- skepticism and misinterpretation of data on public health priorities and benefits
- an "information vacuum" on public health issues
- conflicting values between public health positions on some issues and those of churches and community groups

- concern about the intrusiveness of lifestyle messages
- resentment of public health's regulatory role
- generic antigovernment sentiment; a feeling that public health is yet another waste of tax dollars

Although these responses confirm why public health is so often referred to as a "silent miracle", analysis of the focus-group interviews also yielded several encouraging themes:

- Appreciation for public health's role can be readily stimulated—that is, public health functions that are taken for granted (like clean water, environmental protection, and immunizations) are appreciated once an effort has been made to point out the benefits.
- If informed, people will acknowledge that they benefit from public health, even if they never set foot in the health department.
- Like politics, public health is local. Therefore, when looking for a compelling example of the benefits and value of good public health, look to your own backyard first for those examples.
- Even though they may be resistant to the regulatory roles of public health, people understand that public health regulations are indeed protective and reassuring.

The information about the specific misperceptions some people hold, combined with the insight that there are indeed ways to address those misperceptions, led to the formulation of some key "message concepts" that were most likely to enlighten community members about the importance and value of public health. These include:

- **Public health works.** Such messages highlight public health's many accomplishments and counters negative views of wasteful, ineffective bureaucracies. Public health is cost effective.
- **Prevention works and is a good investment.** Prevention services encompass everything from immunization to health education to restaurant inspections that prevent food-borne pathogens. When we invest, we want two things: profit and value. An investment in health improvement that emphasizes prevention will achieve both. Profit will manifest itself in the productivity and improved quality of life. Value will be created because for a large portion of contemporary health problems, effective prevention yields positive health outcomes at less cost than that of awaiting treatment.[4]
- **Public health protects you and your family.** This concept highlights the fact that public health offers confidence in daily life—that food and water are safe, that new diseases will be detected and countered, that accurate information on health and environmental issues will be

available. Thus public health is for everyone, not just the poor and disadvantaged who are in need of special medical services.

- **Only public health has a mandate to address the health of everyone in your community.** This message reinforces the protective aspect of public health and applies to entire communities as well as to individuals and families. This message concept also captures the unique role of public health in monitoring health status and documenting progress in combating diseases, injuries, and disabilities.

- **Public health is always there.** During disasters, the public turns to public health. Public health's emergency-response role, while sporadic and not applicable in every community, is reassuring and highlights many of public health's otherwise invisible features: rapid response, accurate information, setting priorities, looking out for the community's interests, and preventing disease, to name a few.

- **Public health is indispensable.** Without public health, our quality of life would be palpably worse. We would lose confidence in the safety of our environment and would feel more vulnerable to preventable diseases. We would not know as much about the health status of our communities, nor would we have the information and expertise to address health problems. Without public health, the costs of treating medical conditions, which already account for most of our health care expenditures, would increase even faster.

These message concepts, when applied as a part of a health communications and media advocacy strategy, increase the likelihood of getting public health on your community's map.

A Cautionary Note: Attitudes and perceptions about public health and health promotion will vary across communities. Therefore, before undertaking any of the tactical options described, practitioners should think strategically and follow the same careful diagnostic procedures that have been emphasized throughout this book.

Getting the public health message out is complicated by the reality that, to be effective, you need to reach several audiences with your message.[5] To better manage that complexity, we have found the following process to be helpful. First, delineate all of the possible audiences you need to reach. To help you think strategically, choose one of those audiences. Once you have determined your target audience, answers to the following questions will generate the information that will keep you on track.

How does the target audience perceive public health?

Given the audience's perception, what ideas/benefits do I want to communicate?

What objective do I want to achieve?

What materials do I need to achieve the objective?

Repeat the same process for all of the target audiences you plan to reach. For example, suppose that one of your key audiences is state legislators or county commissioners. By interviewing some of them and/or obtaining information from their voting records, media interviews, or other published statements, you could develop answers to these four questions. Possible answers are provided in Table 4.1.

Following are some ideas that practitioners can consider as they implement a public-awareness campaign.

Strategy 1: Develop and Nurture Relationships with Management and Editorial Staff in the Local Media

Tactic 1.1. Invite reporters, key management, and editorial staff from local media to brown-bag lunches, workshops, and meetings that highlight late-breaking public health issues, key programs, or progress reports.

Tactic 1.2. Take the time to meet with representatives from the media in your community and determine what motivates them and what specific needs they have that public health practitioners can help fulfill. This action responds to the point that Adam Solomon made in the case story: The media do not have a *de facto* responsibility to promote public health.

Tactic 1.3. Promote the development of designated health department staff as expert consultants to contact when media wants to report on a local public health crisis (*e.g.,* an infectious disease outbreak) or to localize a national public health story.

Tactic 1.4. Help practitioners to portray public health as a system by encouraging them to show how various public health activities are interdependent. For example, if a health department is asked to describe its immunization program, public health workers can show continuity by explaining (1) how assessment activities are essential for monitoring trends in the cases of measles in the community; (2) how policies based on disease surveillance ensure timely vaccination of children; (3) how the health department assures the availability of immunization services and vaccines; and (4) how high rates of immunization coverage result not only in preventing disease but also increasing the likelihood that children will be able to experience the social and educational benefits of attending school.

Strategy 2: Implement a Training Program to Enhance Practitioners' Skills in Media Advocacy

Tactic 2.1. Meet with the leader of your local health department to get support to create and manage a series of seminars designed to orient community public health leaders, practitioners, and public health advocates in the process of media advocacy.[6]

TABLE 4.1 Communications Planning Matrix

Audience-Specific Problems/Misconceptions	Communication Objective(s)	Concepts/Materials	Benefits Perceived By Audience
Legislators/County Commissioners • Limited awareness of public health's scope • Antibureaucratic, antiregulatory sentiment • Skepticism toward cost-benefit and other data • "Values" conflict	• Increase sense of public health's relevance and importance • Increase appreciation for positive regulatory role (clean water, safe food), cost-effectiveness and efficiency of public health services • Highlight "neutral" activities that benefit the community at large	• Responsibility for the community's health ("Day in the Life") • Public health works: cost-benefit tied to legislator's interests and a human story • "Day in the Life" and other local examples ("did you know that . . . ?") • Health status report card	• Public health affects me and my constituents, not just "them" • Public health is a worthwhile investment • It's more than condoms in schools, needle exchange, etc. Life would be more dangerous, unpleasant, uncertain, etc. without these services
Boards of Health • Where public health fits in the spectrum of community health services	• Support public health with media, legislators, public	• Cost-benefit information on prevention activities • Health status report	• Public health is a major contributor to our community's health
Managed Care Organizations • Turf issues: Who will be responsible for which services under health reform? • With universal coverage, public health may not be needed	• Partnership with public health to support prevention goals and share data relevant to community health	• Cost-benefit information • Health status report • Unique public health contributions/expertise (e.g., outreach)	• Public health is a key partner for our organization • Public health plays an essential role beyond service provision

Media			
• Perception that public health topics are boring to readers/viewers/listeners • Limited awareness • Public health is clinics for the poor • Public health may no longer be necessary after health care reform	• Increase knowledge and understanding of essential services • Increase awareness of public health's contributions to community health • Increase appreciation for cost-benefit of investment in public health	• "Day in the Life" • Scenarios: what would happen in our community without public health? • Health status report card • "Investigative" angle: investments in prenatal care, TB outreach, or AIDS counseling saved X, but funding is being cut	• Public health is interesting and relevant to me and to my viewers • Public health has a human angle • A strong public health system is essential; the media have a role in covering this topic and reminding legislators of its importance

General Public			
• Limited awareness • Public health is only for poor people; it does not apply to me • Public health is a wasteful bureaucracy • Public health is trying to tell me how to live my life	• Increase awareness of scope and benefits • Show public health's efficiency in its own right, and compared to other expenditures • Demonstrate benefits of public health lifestyle messages	• "Day in the Life" • Public health works • Spokespersons for public health—"What it does for me" • Scenarios—without public health, what would happen?	• Public health protects and serves me, whether I use the health department or not • My family and I need a strong public health system

* "A Day in the Life of Public Health" is a one-page narrative describing the many ways a typical middle-class person benefits from public health—without ever setting foot in the health department. It was developed in 1993 by the Colorado Department of Health.

Tactic 2.2.   Develop the curriculum with a primary emphasis on (1) reframing public debate to increase public support for more effective policy-level approaches to public health problems, and (2) fostering the media's role in setting the public agenda and stimulating public discussion around public health issues.

Tactic 2.3.   Develop practical skill-building sessions where participants can learn and practice how to (1) apply "creative epidemiology," (2) "frame" issues, and (3) gain access to media outlets.

Strategy 3: With Your Community or Service Area, Participate in National Public Health Week to Highlight the Significance of Public Health to the Health of Your Community, State, and Nation

(*Note:* The first week in April has been designated as National Public Health Week in the United States. By adopting a public health week in your community, especially one that coincides with a state or national event, you increase opportunity for positive exposure and promotion of public health and prevention.)

Tactic 3.1.   Work with public health leaders in your community to encourage local government officials to formally declare that one week per year be designated Public Health Week. If possible, the date should coincide with national efforts in order to gain from their promotional and media benefits.

Tactic 3.2.   Establish a Public Health Week consortium of organizations that support the principles of public health—such a consortium would include local print and electronic media, volunteer organizations, hospitals, managed-care groups,insurance companies, public schools, libraries, service clubs, athletic and sports organizations, and businesses.

Tactic 3.3.   Practitioners in the United States should contact the National Association of County and City Health Officials (NACCHO) and request their Health Day Starter Kit. This kit contains sample governmental proclamations, message ideas, and promotional materials, along with tips on activities to highlight during the week.

Strategy 4: Make the Public Aware that Public Health Services are Essential

Tactic 4.1.   Have an inspector take local media or community representatives along on inspections of child-care centers to illustrate the role of essential services in maintaining safe facilities for the community's children.

Strategy 5: Make Data Understandable and More Relevant

Tactic 5.1.   Meet with the health reporter of your local newspaper and offer to generate analyses of health data that he or she can put can put into a periodic "Health Factoid" feature (as appears in *USA Today*, for example).

Tactic 5.2.   Hold a data-sharing seminar with other organizations indicating that your data may be used by their organizations to develop programs and plan activities.

Tactic 5.3.   Be prepared to take advantage of opportunities to discuss local or state data when a national survey on a health issue hits the press.

Tactic 5.4.   Publish a comprehensive report card on the health status of the community that includes specific indicators, essential services conducted to derive that data, the specific division of the health department responsible for those indicators, and any other services and/or programs that address those indicators.

Tactic 5.5.   A story reporting a severe health problem or disease outbreak in another area or county can provide a timely opportunity to educate citizens in your community about the essential protective services your health department provides. For example, if an outbreak of a waterborne disease is reported in a nearby city, your local media may find it newsworthy to publish a story asking: "How Safe Are We Here?" If justified, such a story could be a key vehicle to inform the public why their support for a public health infrastructure has value.

Strategy 6: Reach the Decision Makers

Tactic 6.1.   With fellow public health advocates, adopt a decision maker![7] Make contact and establish a relationship. If the decision maker in question is a legislator, your best chances to make contact are likely to be through a staff member. Listen to the decision maker and pay attention. Find out what he or she knows and believes about health. Become the decision maker's resource and expert on public health issues. If such a relationship is viewed to be too political, work with other advocates to fill such a role: university professors, graduate students, retired former health workers, and members of volunteer health organizations.

Tactic 6.2.   Sponsor conferences or seminars on public and community health for decision makers and practitioners. Such conferences create opportunities for interaction between public health practitioners and state legislators. Meals and social gatherings at these events provide an informal setting for learning and exchanging ideas.

Tactic 6.3. Examine the evaluations you have made of your health promotion and disease prevention programs. Where you have the data, use cost-effectiveness and cost-benefit analysis to show program value and comparative savings. When using data, never forget the faces that represent those numbers.

PARTICIPATION

The word *participate* means to share or take part with others in some activity or enterprise. With regard to health promotion activities and programs, we think it is useful to think of community participation as having two complementary dimensions. One refers to the participation of multiple organizations in the planning and delivery of health promotion programs; the other refers to circumstances where community members are seen not merely as recipients of a program, but as active participants in shaping and implementing that program.

In this section, we emphasize the latter point. In doing so, however, we offer practitioners two cautions:

Caution 1: Do not minimize the importance of reaching out and establishing partnerships with organizations and groups whose participation can enhance your efforts to improve the health of the community you serve. It goes without saying that a local health department would be in for a rude awakening if it tried to launch a breast cancer screening program without coordinating with its local volunteer cancer agency and local physicians.

Caution 2: We all understand that heavy-handed, expert-only decision making in communities is a formula for disaster. At the same time, the need to enhance citizen participation should not be mistaken as a call for practitioners to apologize for their training and experience and abdicate their professional skills and knowledge. The enemies of true participation are those who create divisiveness by their relentless pursuit of the "right" answer or the "right" way. Convergence of differing points will result from a combination of common courtesy, listening, and a genuine desire to achieve something better. Our best advice is simple: Don't use "listening" as a tactic and then "lay on" your expertise. Listen to learn, and then be honest in your own response. Recall Ray Wycoff's experience in Greene County. The planning team had reasonable representation from multiple organizations, and did come up with a scientifically sound program idea. But even though their interorganizational and scientific ducks seemed to be in order, their failure to take into account the values and interests of the individuals they were trying to reach led to difficulties.

Why Is Participation Important?

Consider the nature of the problems practitioners work on and the context in which they address them. Over the years, findings from epidemiologic and behavioral research have given us a better understanding of the events and circumstances that seem to shape and even predict the preventable problems you are likely to face in your community: heart disease, cancer, injuries, suicide, homicide, alcohol and drug abuse, teen pregnancy, preventable problems associated with aging, AIDS, and so on. The events and circumstances that explain the occurrence of these health problems are often expressed as a causal chain.

In theory, if you know the elements of the causal chain and can modify them, chances are that you can prevent the problem in question. But the term *causal chain* paints a deceptive picture of linear order. In reality, it is a very messy, convoluted chain! It is a mixture of biological, behavioral, environmental, political, and economic factors.

Furthermore, few if any of these factors are stable; not only will they vary in degree over time, they will also vary from country to country, state to state, province to province, community to community, neighborhood to neighborhood, and so on. Given the inevitability that practitioners must address complex, moving targets, it is safe to say that programs and policies aimed at preventing such problems are not likely to be effective without the informed, active involvement of individuals, families, and local groups and institutions; this is especially true when one tries to undertake a public-policy or legislative approach to health promotion or disease prevention.

No doubt there are many of us who can identify with Ray Wycoff's experience in Greene County: the gnawing truth that we failed to engage people who should have been involved. Based on our experience, we believe that such failure is most often the result of an unintended error of omission, caused primarily because the practitioner loses sight of the principle of participation.[8]

Of all the concepts that help shape research and practice in community health promotion, none generates more consensus than the citizen dimension of community participation. This frequently cited passage from the 1974 Alma Ata Declaration captures not only the intent of the concept, but its relevance and ethic as well: "...people have the right and the duty to participate individually and collectively in the planning and implementing of their health care."[9]

A well-trained, talented, and experienced person is capable of solving problems and overcoming challenges that might baffle others who are less talented and experienced. In many jobs, talented people can carry out their work with minimal or no involvement of those who receive their services. Examples include the expert plumber, microbiologist, auto mechanic, chemist, or tailor. Such is not the case for capable community health promotion practitioners; a key element of their competency is the capacity to engage community members and elicit their participation in all phases of their work: planning, implementation, and evaluation. This element of community participation must be an integral part of the practitioner's *mental model.*

In 1986, Lawrence Green proposed a set of propositions for the purpose of validating theories of participation.[10] We have modified these propositions and offer them up as a means to test your own mental model with respect to participation. As you read each of the four propositions below, simply ask yourself, "To what extent is this statement consistent with my own beliefs?"

1. As the level of active—as opposed to passive—participation of the people in the planning and implementation process increases, the probability of achieving health improvement goals will also increase.
2. Both active participation and consensus will increase as people are engaged, listened to, and informed about community health status and opportunities for health improvement.
3. As people receive feedback on the progress of programs and services they have had a hand in shaping, their trust and participation will increase.

Editorial squabbles aside, community health promotion practitioners who have difficulty acting on these propositions are likely to repeat the experiences Ray Wycoff had in Greene County.

When practitioners think about engaging the community, one of the first things to come to mind is the notion of a community coalition—a group of people representative of a community, coalesced by the shared interest to achieve a common vision. For example, the community of Atlanta formed a coalition whose goal was to secure the 1996 Olympic Games. The success of that coalition is testimony to common sense: dictatorships aside, representative groups can accomplish what one person cannot.

Assembling a coalition or working group is one thing; managing and keeping that group on track is another. Even with the best of intentions, problems can arise that disrupt or even destroy the spirit of cooperative group process. If practitioners are sensitive and alert to these problems, the majority of problems can be prevented or at least minimized.

Following are examples of four problems that commonly come to the surface. We express these problems as symptoms and give examples of how those symptoms surface in day-to-day practice. We then suggest steps that might be taken to address those symptoms or to prevent them from arising. As you read through the examples, keep in mind that healthy, productive coalitions are never free of conflict; problems and disagreements are inherent and often beneficial in the robust planning process. The challenge is to anticipate and prevent unnecessary problems and manage disagreement and conflict.

Symptom #1: Members of organizations not included in the planning activities resist your planning process and proposals.

Example.   A group of physicians who have been working on mammography screening have not been consulted by your group as you develop plans for a more comprehensive cancer prevention program. As your group presents its plan for funding and support, the physician group gets word to key decision-makers that the resources in question would be more efficiently spent on their specific mammography program. With such input from a reputable group, the decision-makers are likely to put your request for support on hold until some clarification is achieved.

Tactic.   To minimize the chance of such opposition, place a priority (early on and throughout the planning process) on notifying and querying all parties and organizations that might have an interest or an investment in some aspect of the issue or problem you plan to address. This can be accomplished by taking the following action steps:

1. Ask all persons involved in the initiation of the planning to identify organizations or individuals who may have an interest or stake in the issue at hand. Planning group members should be encouraged to make personal contact with those organizations or individuals to inform them of your intentions and to determine their level of interest.

2. Develop written communications (newsletters, memos, electronic mail) and diffuse them through existing community channels.

3. Develop and implement a policy to make formal announcements in public meetings or mass media channels. In all communications, include a request for inquiries and ideas.

Symptom #2: The coalition's business is disrupted by members of the group who argue about the direction that is being taken; competing agendas become problematic.

Example.   A member of the planning group is most adamant about moving as quickly as possible to the implementation of a cervical cancer screening program for a low-income population because "the problem is evident." This person has expressed strong opposition to recommendations of the health department representative who has been urging the group to give priority to an epidemiologic analysis of women's health problems, which has not yet been done for the proposed target area. The conflict is a classic case of "it needs further study" versus "we need to act now."

Tactic.   Because such spirited differences are commonplace, we encourage leaders to view such moments as opportunities for growth. Consider these actions:

- Early in the process of selection of members of the planning team, ask members to (1) declare the mission of their agency or organization, or the bias they bring as an unaffiliated member; (2) indicate how the "vision" the planning group seeks is related to their mission or personal bias. Indicate to them what roles they will and will not be permitted to play.

- When conflict arises over vested interests, encourage the relevant parties to reexamine the vision and mission statements and use those as a means to return their discussion to common ground. In the case of the illustration given, the point should be made that both goals have merit. Help resolve the conflict by assisting in a reframing of the problem. Rather than debating the merits of program versus data collection and analysis, the question should be: How can we have useful data without depleting needed program resources and unduly delaying implementation? Keep everyone focused on the vision.

Symptom #3: Participation in the coalition declines and becomes limited to a small group representing a narrow range of interest, often accompanied by reports of "burnout."

Example.   There is high turnout and great enthusiasm during the first two planning meetings. Then, with each subsequent meeting, you notice a steady decline in attendance. A small core of participants maintains the burden. There is talk of burnout and attendance becomes sporadic. In retrospect, you found it easy to form the planning group but difficult to maintain it.

Tactic.   Depending on the circumstances, it may take a year to complete the planning process. It is unrealistic to expect people, who are already busy and committed to their day-to-day routines, to have the time and energy to stay with a long and demanding planning process. Following are strategic steps to increase planning efficiency and keep the time burden manageable for members of the planning team:

- In your first meeting, use clear, concise agendas designed to address the highest priority issues. Indicate that there will be few large-group meetings; those that are held will be kept short.

- Distribute and manage the tasks. Planning group members have varied interests. Determine their special areas of interest and form small "task groups" based on those interests. Through the collective input of the planning group in early meetings, delineate specific activities for the respective task groups and determine when, in the course of the planning process, the product of their activity is due.

- This small task group approach will help maintain the integrity of the planning team by allowing members (1) to move in and out of the planning process as their expertise is needed, thus reducing the time burden; and (2) to focus on issues most closely associated with their priorities and expertise.
- Develop a Gannt chart, showing which tasks are due at what time; make this chart available to all members of the planning team.
- To keep all members informed of key issues and progress, publish a planning team communiqué, or newsletter at regular intervals.

Symptom #4: Actions and intentions of the planning group or coalition are misrepresented either in the media or in public discussions.

Example.   As a result of your planning process, comprehensive school health education has emerged as a key element for a proposed community health promotion program. Your group is surprised when an article appears in the newspaper revealing that a group of "concerned citizens" is alarmed because your proposal for comprehensive school health is really a cover for a liberal "sex education" program. The article is followed by TV news coverage, and various agency cosponsors involved in the planning receive queries. Many people start asking, "What's going on?"

Action.   Early in the planning process, set aside specific time to anticipate efforts by those who would try to misrepresent your intentions. Continually ask questions like: Who needs to be informed of our activities? and How might a given activity be misinterpreted? Develop a strategy to keep all members of the planning team (and the key decision-makers in the organizations they represent) routinely informed. Any one, or a combination, of the following techniques, will promote such awareness: (1) a regular newsletter, (2) periodic briefing or update sessions, or (3) special memos alerting relevant parties of key or potentially controversial issues. Establish a liaison with representatives from the local print and electronic media (it is ideal to have a media person on the planning team). News items on key issues and outcomes of the planning process not only increase the visibility of the proposed program and heighten public awareness, they also serve to reinforce the significance of the planning process in the eyes of the planning team members.

Tactics to Engage "Plain Folks."   The wisdom of coalitions is all around us. Globally there are few nationally funded health promotion initiatives or demonstrations that do not require evidence that some form of coalition has been established to ensure community collaboration. While we applaud and support such policy, the fact remains that Ray Wycoff's failure to expand his planning group beyond representatives of official agencies to include "plain folks" is not as rare as one would hope. Frankly, it is easier to pick up the phone and get the commitment of people who are already devoted to the issue at hand. And why not? It is part of their job, and they may get some added resources; in short, they have a built-in incentive. Getting "plain folks" to participate is a lot tougher, and it takes a precious commodity we seem to have very little of: time. But sometimes the answers to difficult problems are not as complicated as we make them. The following tactics serve to illustrate this point.

Tactic 1. Gather information about the population, or populations, your program is supposed to serve. Where do you start? Suppose you are traveling across the country and your car breaks down on a Friday night in an area you know nothing about. You're told your car can't be fixed until Monday afternoon or Tuesday. In addition to "asking around," one of the fastest ways to find out something about the place you're in is to scan the local newspaper. Whether it is a monthly, weekly, or daily publication, it will give you a good deal of insight about the place through news features, announcements, a calendar of events, and advertisements.

The extent to which one learns about a community is largely dependent upon the desire to do so, as we saw when Ray Wycoff drove out to see Reverend Carver. The point here is that practitioners need to drive out to meet their Reverend Carvers *before* being shamed into doing so. As a health promotion practitioner, you may have access to existing records and data sources. If so, you should use them to create a demographic and epidemiologic profile that will help you sharpen your picture of the people and their community.

Tactic 2. Once you feel you have a reasonable understanding of the community, get out into it! In some instances, especially where racial, cultural, and ethnic diversity come into play, your most appropriate entrée to the community may be through indigenous leaders or "gatekeepers" (neighborhood leaders, local service providers, business owners, clergy, youth workers, teachers, senior citizen workers). As Ron Braithwaite and his colleagues have astutely observed, in some instances you should prepare for a "period of suspicion."[11] Sadly, the experience in many minority or under-served communities has been one of unkept promises and disappointments—and such histories are not easily forgotten. It takes time to establish the reciprocal trust required to build a partnership. *NOTE:* Too often we make the error of underestimating the time it takes to establish community rapport and trust.

Tactic 3. Contact local institutions. Kretzman and McKnight found that local libraries often serve as a central meeting place for many community organizations.[12] The librarian can give you information on groups that meet there, and sometimes libraries keep a self-published directory of local organizations. Besides health-related groups, local organizations to contact might include churches, parks and recreation departments, schools, law enforcement agencies, art or cultural centers, and business associations.

Tactic 4. Apply the awareness tactics spelled out earlier in this chapter to let people in the community know about opportunities for participating in health promotion programs and activities.

Tactic 5. Use incentives and recognition as a part of your efforts to recruit and sustain participation.

Tactic 6. Invite community members to participate in a seminar that highlights key health issues and to share their ideas about those issues. Use such gatherings and events to survey attendees to assess their willingness and interest in participating; identify the skills they have and what roles they might be willing to play as part of an emerging health initiative.

A serious commitment to engaging community members in your work is a direct reflection of respect: a deferential regard to a fellow citizen, the acknowledgment of worth. The following is an excerpt from an essay written by Kentucky essayist Wendell Berry.[13] In this piece, Berry describes meeting a fellow Kentuckian and discovering that they have something in common. We think that Berry's story captures the spirit of community respect and serves as an appropriate transition to the final topic in this chapter: social capital.[14]

"I've heard of Middletown," I said. "It was the home of my father's great friend, John W. Jones."

"Well, John W. Jones was my uncle."

I told him then of my father's and my own respect for Mr. Jones.

"I want to tell you a story about Uncle John," he said. And he told me this:

When his Uncle John was president of the bank in North Middletown, his policy was to give a loan to any graduate of the North Middletown High School who wanted to go to college and needed the money. This practice caused great consternation to the bank examiners who came and found those unsecured loans on the books and no justification for them except Mr. Jones's conviction that it was right to make them.

As it turned out, it was right in more than principle, for in the many years that Mr. Jones was president of the bank, making those "unsound loans," all of the loans were repaid; he never lost a dime on a one of them.

I do not mean to raise here the question of the invariable goodness of a college education, which I doubt. My point in telling this story is that Mr. Jones was acting from a kind of knowledge, inestimably valuable and probably indispensable, that comes out of common culture and that cannot be taught as a part of the formal curriculum of a school . . . what he knew—

and this involved his knowledge of himself, his tradition, his community, and everybody in it—was that trust, in the circumstances then present, could beget trustworthiness. This is the kind of knowledge, obviously, that is fundamental to the possibility of community life and to certain good possibilities in the character of people.

SOCIAL CAPITAL

In 1923, C. E. A. Winslow demonstrated insightful vision when he characterized public health as the science and art of preventing disease, prolonging life, and promoting health and well-being *through organized community efforts* for the sanitation of the environment, the control of communicable infections, the organization of medical and nursing services for the early diagnosis and prevention of disease, the education of the individual in personal health, and the development of the *social machinery* to assure a standard of living adequate for the maintenance and improvement of health.[15]

The two italicized phrases, *through organized community efforts* and *social machinery,* are curiously similar to key elements of a theory that has recently gained prominence globally among scholars in a variety of different fields: the theory of social capital.

In this final section, we describe some of the fundamental ideas behind social capital with the intent of pointing out its potential relevance for health promotion practitioners.

Social capital refers to the process of people and organizations within a community working collaboratively in an atmosphere of trust toward the accomplishment of mutual social benefit. Evidence, especially in the sociological, educational, and political science literature, indicates that the constructs that make up the notion of social capital are measurable. One of the most frequently referenced scholars studying social capital is Robert Putnam, a professor of political science at Harvard.[16] He has defined social capital as the processes among people that establish networks, norms, and social trust, and facilitate coordination and cooperation for mutual benefit.

The foundation for Putnam's ideas about social capital was influenced in part by his study of local governments in Italy from 1970 to 1990.[17] In 1970, a new set of regional governments was established in Italy, all of which, on paper at least, had comparable organizational structures and adequate resources in relative terms. Putnam's research revealed that two decades after the 1970 reorganization, there were some rather dramatic differences among some of the communities. One group of communities was very inefficient—they were corrupt, tended to be managed on the basis of favors to small special-interest groups, and appeared to invest little in civic improvement and development programs. Others, however, operated under more democratic and interdependent principles, and civic programs such as arts and sports groups, day-care centers, industrial parks, job programs, and family clinics were much more visible.

Putnam concluded that the more efficient and effective governments were those where citizens demonstrated high levels of what he termed "civic engagement." Indicators of civic engagement were manifested by rather common acts of social investment: voter turnout, newspaper readership, and participation in cooperative groups such as sporting clubs, parent/teacher organizations, local arts and theater activities, and so on. Putnam observed that central to these civic actions was a sense of social trust.

The critical elements of social capital include the following:

- Trust
- Cooperation/coordination
- Civic engagement
- Reciprocity

What relevance does the concept of social capital have for health promotion? The most obvious link between health promotion and the concept of social capital lies in the reality that community is at the heart of both. We now have ample empirical evidence showing us that effective public health programs do indeed require the effective application of what C. E. A. Winslow referred to as "organized community efforts" and the development and/or activation of a community's "social machinery." Even among community-based health promotion interventions that apply sound theory and methods and have adequate economic resources for implementation, there is considerable variability in the effects of those interventions. We believe that there is sufficient circumstantial evidence to suggest that the presence or absence of social capital within an intervention community may account for some portion of that variability.

If social scientists are correct in assuming that a high level of civic engagement is a true indicator of social capital, then one may logically ask, "To what extent is the level of social capital associated with the acceptance, application, and effectiveness of a community health promotion program?" This in turn gives rise to at least four interesting empirical questions that health promotion researchers and practitioners might ask:

1. Can we define social capital within the context of health promotion?

2. Can we measure social capital in communities?

3. If we can develop valid measures of social capital, is there any evidence that levels of social capital are associated with the level of effectiveness of health promotion programs?

4. If social capital can be measured and found to be associated with the effectiveness of health promotion programs, can it be created or modified?

Answers to these questions will help practitioners understand to what extent the effectiveness of community health promotion programs depends on not only the community's interest in making the "civic investment" needed, but also its capability to do so.

The potential ability to measure social capital creates the opportunity to assess a community's level of readiness for the application of health promotion programs, which depends upon the activation and support of social networks. In turn, this may enable us to describe the elusive notion of "empowerment" in more specific terms and, more important, to legitimize planned social and community development as a valid and fundable component of community health promotion.

For example, on the matter of whether or not social capital is measurable, a large number of community psychologists, social epidemiologists, social scientists, and community health promotion researchers are already studying various dimensions of social capital.[18] Eng and Parker have developed an assessment tool consisting of eight interrelated dimensions; they call the collective measure "community competence." Buckner has developed an instrument that provides a valid means of assessing the perceived cohesion in a given neighborhood. Wickizer and his colleagues have developed and tested a technique to measure the extent to which community health promotion programs cause the formation and operation of tangible social networks and whether these networks tend to predict change. Fawcett and his co-workers have developed a practical method for tracking events and changes in a community's system and linking those to changes in selected measures of health. This latter technique may indeed provide some evidence that properly administered community health promotion programs may contribute to the creation of social capital.

It is possible that social capital may not only be an important explanatory factor (independent variable) in the evaluation of the effectiveness of health promotion programs, but that social capital may also be an outcome (dependent variable) generated by the implementation of effective community health promotion interventions.

SUMMARY

As the millennium approaches, we anticipate increasing theory development and applied research activity focusing on the political, social, and economic determinants of health.[19] Some of this activity will include further exploration of how social capital influences the effectiveness of community-based efforts to improve health. Regardless of what specific directions these inquiries follow, it is likely that community-based participatory research will be employed as a principal methodologic strategy. Such approaches require a huge amount of carefully planned, culturally sensitive fieldwork. Health promotion practitioners, with their practical experience and sense of social connectedness, are well positioned to play an important role in this kind of research. How well that role is played out will depend in part upon the extent to which practitioners have a working knowledge of the concepts presented in this chapter.

ENDNOTES

1. Dall T. *Political Theory and Praxis.* Minneapolis: University of Minnesota Press; 1977.
2. Rose G. *The Strategy of Preventive Medicine.* New York: Oxford University Press; 1992:123. In this classic 125-page paperback, the late Professor Rose combines his command of science with his sensitive humanity to give public health workers insights they can apply every day. We think it should be a part of every practitioner's personal library.
3. *Marketing Core Public Health Functions: Summary of Focus Group Findings and Implications for Message Concepts.* Macro International, Inc., and Westat Inc., August 1994. Contract study with the Centers for Disease Control and Prevention #200-93-0653. Practitioners will find this straightforward description a useful resource.
4. Tolsma DD, Koplan JP. Health behaviors and health promotion. In: Last JM, Wallace RB, eds. *Public Health and Preventive Medicine.* 13th ed. East Norwalk, CT: Appleton and Lange; 1992:701–714.
5. Paradoxically, the complexity of multiple audiences is also one of your strongest assets, since it gives you a broader and more diverse base of support that decreases the perception of self-interest. Multiple audiences constitute an advantage to be treasured.
6. As a first point of departure in preparing the plan and content for the seminars, we recommend two rich sources of information: Wallack L, Dorfman L, Jernigan D, Themba M. *Media Advocacy and Public Health.* Newbury Park, CA: Sage Publications; 1993; and Chapman S, Lupton D. *The Fight for Public Health: Principles and Practice of Media Advocacy.* London: BMJ Publishing; 1994.
7. By *decision makers,* we generally mean people who are elected or appointed to government positions such as neighborhood or city councils, boards of county commissioners, and legislatures.
8. For an in-depth and well-referenced discussion on the principle of participation, see Green L. Theory of participation: a qualitative analysis of its expression in national and international health policies. In: Ward WB, ed. *Advances in Health Education and Promotion.* Greenwich, CT: JAI Press Inc.; 1986: 1(part A):211–236.
9. World Health Organization. Alma-Ata 1978: *Primary Health Care.* Geneva: World Health Organization, "Health for All" Series No. 1.
10. The four propositions presented here have been modified for application in this text from a longer list of propositions offered by Lawrence Green in the reference cited in endnote 8.
11. Braithwaite R, Murphy F, Lythcott N, Blumenthal D. Community organization and development for health promotion within an urban black community: a conceptual model. *Health Educ.* 1989;20(5):56–60.

12. Kretzman J, McKnight J. *Building Communities from the Inside Out.* Chicago: ACTA Publications; 1993.
13. Berry W. *What Are People For?* New York: North Point Press; 1990:118–119.
14. Although Robert Putnam is widely cited for his work on the subject of social capital, Putnam himself attributes the development of the theoretical framework for social capital to James S. Coleman.
15. Winslow CEA. *The Evolution and Significance of the Modern Public Health Campaign.* New Haven, CT: Yale University Press; 1923. (Reprinted in 1984 by the Journal of Public Health Policy.)
16. Putnam R. The prosperous community: social capital and public life. *American Prospect,* 1993;143:35–42.
17. Putnam R. *Making Democracy Work: Civic Traditions in Modern Italy.* Princeton, NJ: Princeton University Press; 1993.
18. The work of these researchers represents only a portion of the work which attempts to measure various dimensions of social capital. The references mentioned in the text are: Eng E, Parker E. Measuring community competence in the Mississippi Delta: the interface between program evaluation and empowerment. *Health Educ Q.* 1994;21(2):199–220; Buckner J. The development of an instrument to measure neighborhood cohesion. *J Comm Psychology.* 1988;16(6):771–790; and Wickizer T, VonKorff M, Cheadle A, et al. Activating communities for health promotion: a process of evaluation method. *Am J Public Health.* 1993;83:561–567. The best and most practical reference for the work of Steve Fawcett and his co-workers is Fawcett S, Francisco W, Paine-Andrews A, et al. *Work Group Evaluation Handbook: Evaluating and Supporting Community Interventions for Health and Development,* published by the Work Group for Health and Community Development, 1486 Dole Center, Kansas University, Lawrence, KS 66045.
19. Marmot M. The Social Pattern of Health and Disease. In: Blane D, Brunner E, and Wilkinson R, eds. *Health and Social Organization.* London: Routledge; 1996.

CHAPTER 5

Theory Applied

Case Story
THE OLD HORSE

His granddaughter called him *Lao Ma* ("old horse") because one of her favorite pastimes was to climb up on his back and ride him around the house. In addition to being an "old horse," he was also known as Dr. Yu Mei, director of the Ministry of Public Health (MOPH) for Zhejiang Province in the People's Republic of China. Dr. Yu was a highly respected public health official in China who had distinguished himself through his pioneering public health work. In 1980, he received international recognition when the World Health Organization (WHO) honored him with a distinguished service medal for his accomplishments in tuberculosis (TB) control. Dr. Yu was an advocate of health education because it had been an essential part of his TB prevention and control efforts.

The literal English translation of the Chinese expression for the term *health education* is "health propaganda." This fits the Chinese tradition of public campaigns that used banners, posters, pamphlets, and community lectures to communicate health messages. The central government had established an entity called the National Patriotic Health Campaign Committee (NPHCC) to provide national health education leadership; virtually all communities in China have a local NPHCC.

Like many of his Chinese public health colleagues, Dr. Yu was well aware that his country was experiencing a health transition: better control of communicable and infectious diseases meant that more people would survive to adulthood, which in turn meant that more persons would be at risk for chronic health problems like heart disease, stroke, and cancers. Dr. Yu knew that the disturbing smoking trends in China made this pattern of transition more problematic. Virtually all of the surveys on tobacco use showed that nearly 70 percent of all men in China smoke. And, although the surveys indicated that few women in China are smokers, there was an increase in smoking among younger women, especially in the larger cities. Dr. Yu was also aware that as China continued to move ahead as a market-driven economy, its health profile would surely begin to reflect those of some other market economies, including both the positive and negative effects of market forces.

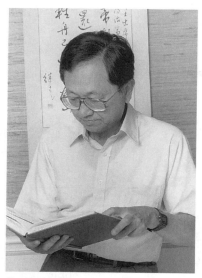

Dr. Yu Mei

Because of his expertise in tuberculosis prevention, Dr. Yu was a frequent consultant to WHO in Geneva. It was through his contact with WHO that he became aware of the health education and health promotion innovations that were emerging in areas of public health other than TB; he viewed the cardiovascular risk-reduction programs in Europe, Scandinavia, Canada, Australia, and the United States with keen interest. These programs were more complex and went beyond the traditional Chinese approach to health education; Dr. Yu was eager to experiment with these Western methods to see if they could be adapted as part of the prevention strategy in his health ministry.

Dr. Yu was especially interested in the community intervention work being carried out by Dr. Pekka Puska and his co-workers in Finland. As Dr. Yu developed long-range prevention plans for his province, he frequently sought the counsel of Dr. Puska.

Dr. Li Fang (pronounced "Lee Fong") had completed her medical training at Shanghai Medical University and had stayed on for an additional year of studies in public health. Her dream to return to her home province to practice public health was realized in January when she accepted an offer from Dr. Yu to become the health education coordinator for the Zhejiang Province MOPH.

In some regions of China it is customary for friends and co-workers, especially when speaking informally, to refer to younger persons by placing the word *shao* before their names. So, outside of formal circles, with courtesy and respect, Dr. Li Fang was called *Shao Fang*. In Shao Fang, Dr. Yu was hopeful that he had found the person who could take the leadership in implementing a new vision of health education and health promotion in Zhejiang Province.

During her first six-months on the job, Shao Fang spent the majority of her time working alongside co-workers from other units of the MOPH as a part of the MOPH planning team. Their task was to prepare the Provincial Health Plan for the Year 2000, modeled in part after the WHO Health for All by the Year 2000 documents and Healthy People 2000, a health promotion/disease prevention planning document developed in the United States.

Shao Fang and her colleagues pored through mounds of data and reports. They looked at patterns and trends of health problems and risk factors, then examined those patterns against the usual social, economic, educational, and employment variables. As they began to identify high-priority problems and formulate health objectives, there was no denying that the problem of tobacco consumption was huge. Data on smoking and health in China was shocking: World Bank studies showed that tobacco was causing about half a million deaths a year in China, half of which were from chronic lung disease. Left unchecked, the rate of tobacco consumption among men (70 percent) would lead to an epidemic of unnecessary chronic diseases; it would cause premature death and disability that would, by 2020 or 2030, have the joint effect of diminishing the work-

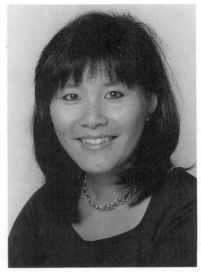

Dr. Li Fang

force and crippling the Chinese system of health. The chilling reality about this effect was not whether, but precisely when, it would occur.

In May, after members of the MOPH advisory council had reviewed a working draft of the Provincial Health Plan for the Year 2000, Dr. Yu announced that tobacco-use prevention and control was to be one of the top health priorities for the MOPH. He also announced that he was assigning Shao Fang to take the lead in developing an anti-tobacco demonstration project for one of the communities within the province. He needed to show that a planned tobacco-use prevention and control program was feasible and could be effective. Once he was able to show effectiveness and feasibility, dissemination throughout the province, and perhaps to the rest of China, would follow.

Dr. Yu informed Shao Fang that he would make arrangements for her to participate in the upcoming annual two-week community-intervention training course held by Dr. Puska and his colleagues in early July at Joensuu, North Karelia, Finland. The announcement for the training course indicated that there would be several experts there who had developed tobacco-use control programs in other countries; the timing couldn't have been better. Shao Fang's excitement about the trip was tempered by the reality that she was undertaking a large responsibility and had much to accomplish before leaving for Finland.

The Eastern District of the city of Hangzhou was chosen as the demonstration site. Shao Fang's initial first step was to assemble a planning group; it was aptly called the No-Smoking Team. First she got the support and participation of the local Patriotic Health Campaign Committee and successfully recruited key representatives from hospitals, schools, businesses, volunteer cancer agencies, and the media.

With the support and counsel of Dr. Yu, the No-Smoking Team was able to secure the participation of two of the Eastern District's key political figures. The planning process was underway.

*   *   *

In July, northern Finland is the land of the midnight sun. Shao Fang was taken by the fact that the sun never seemed to set; it turned out to be quite appropriate, though, because she was far more interested in exploring new ideas than sleeping! She had read most of the literature published on the cardiovascular community-intervention trials and had a good general understanding of the process. What she wanted out of the training was more detail, especially about the methods and the thinking that led to those methods. She framed all of her questions in terms of the tobacco-use prevention and control task she and her co-workers in the Eastern District of Hangzhou had in front of them. New information and interesting ideas were everywhere—but two concepts stood out for Shao Fang.

The first had to do with school health education. She and members of the No-Smoking Team had recognized that schools were likely to play a major role in whatever program emerged. What she learned in the training was that with thoughtful planning, schools could serve as an effective means to reach and engage the support of parents. One of the visiting faculty members, Dr. Cheryl Perry from Minnesota, presented evidence from her work in Minnesota and other American programs that school-based approaches could have an influence upon specific health habits of parents.

The second was a theory that suggested that individual human health behavior changes in accordance to the extent to which an individual is more or less ready to change. Appropriately called *Stages of Change Model,* this theory sets forth the proposition that behavior change is not a single event, but a series of events that depend upon an individual's readiness to change. According to this theory, there are five different levels of readiness to make and sustain changes.

The names of the stages are almost self-explanatory. For example, the stage in which a person is furthest from attempting a change is called the *precontemplation* stage; the next stage is *contemplation*; then comes the *ready for action* or *decision* stage, followed by the *action* stage. The final stage is called *maintenance.*

As Shao Fang thought more about this theory, it seemed clear that there were real possibilities for its application in the tobacco-use prevention and control program she and her colleagues were planning. She thought to herself: *If a large number of men in the Eastern District are not in the* ready for action *stage, a large campaign on smoking cessation may not be a good investment of time and effort!*

She also learned that numerous studies in the United States had used standardized questions in surveys to determine the distribution of levels of readiness to change within populations—so not only was it possible to measure these so-called Stages of Change in a population of smokers, but it was also possible to detect whether changes occur in the stages over time. Dr. Yu was unambiguous about the issue of evaluation; he had made repeated references to his desire to see some evidence of program effects.

Shao Fang had much to share with her colleagues back in Hangzhou.

*   *   *

Twenty people were seated around the long table, which was dotted with cups containing loose ground tea, large Thermos jugs full of piping hot water, and small bowls of fresh fruit. Senior staff from the Zhejiang Province MOPH were joined by members of the No-Smoking Team; no one was more eager to hear Shao Fang's debriefing report than Dr. Yu.

She began with a few slides of the Joensuu countryside. "This is a picture of our hotel at 12 noon; this is our hotel at 3 A.M. As you can see, no difference!" The chuckle was polite.

After providing a brief summary of the content covered in the training program, Shao Fang began to describe how the No-Smoking Team members could strengthen their school health approach by adding a specific component designed to reach parents. She then shifted attention to the possible application of Stages of Change theory. She explained how, by incorporating just a few questions into their baseline survey, they could get two benefits: (1) some valuable information to help them plan their intervention, and (2) data showing whether their program caused a shift in the population of men's readiness to quit smoking.

Dr. Yu sat back and observed the questions and discussion that Shao Fang's report had stimulated. After a most animated and lively exchange, there was consensus that translation of the Stages of Change questions into Chinese would not compromise the construct being measured. Dr. Yu said little.

*   *   *

Baseline surveys were initiated in the middle of August. By October, the No-Smoking Team had the results from the Stages of Change measurements. Approximately 68 percent of the men and 7 percent of the women sampled were regular smokers. Of the men who smoked, 72 percent fell into the precontemplation category. The survey also showed that among youth age thirteen to fifteen, 34 percent of boys and 4 percent of girls reported that they smoked at least occasionally.

Liu Baoyi had been assigned to take the lead in preparing the intervention plan. He had been a part of the health education team for the

MOPH's successful tuberculosis-control program. A popular and well-respected figure in the Eastern District, Liu Baoyi was known more for his accomplishments as the premier football (soccer) coach for young people in the community than for his work with the MOPH.

After getting comments on a first draft of the plan, Liu Baoyi presented the final proposed strategy to the No-Smoking Team on September 1. He explained that they would take a comprehensive approach involving the local cancer society, businesses, and media, as well as the local Patriotic Health Campaign Committee—the focal point for the program was to be the Eastern District school system. The primary components included:

1. A health curriculum that placed emphasis on teaching children about the harmful effects of smoking and was variably tailored for students in grades two through six.

2. A coordinated media campaign wherein the radio, television, and newspapers featured stories and information about the health effects of tobacco.

3. Smoking-cessation self-help clinics promoted and made accessible through the local volunteer cancer organization.

4. A planned effort by local political officials advocating the implementation of policies that promote smoke-free areas in public places and businesses.

He then explained that planning had been influenced by two key points: (1) timing and (2) the application of Stages of Change theory within the context of traditional Chinese cultural beliefs.

Liu Baoyi gave a brief review of the analysis of smoking prevalence and an overview of Stages of Change theory, and concluded by pointing out that the baseline data clearly showed that the majority of male smokers were in the precontemplative Stage of Change.[1]

Then he announced: "Here is our strategy to reach them: May 31 is World No-Tobacco Day and June 1 is Children's Day.[2] Since we know that a large majority of fathers are smokers who are precontemplatives, we have arranged for all the children to bring home a letter to their fathers the day before World No-Tobacco Day. The letter will read:

> Dear Father:
>
> This letter comes from the bottom of my heart.
>
> I have been learning about the harm of smoking in school and my heart is heavy. Science shows us that smoking can cause lung cancer and heart disease and cause death before people get old. Also, the smoke from others can harm those who do not smoke.
>
> It worries me to see you smoke.

As I grow up, I will need your love and wisdom to help me. Tomorrow is "World No-Tobacco Day"; won't you please consider giving up smoking?

The day after tomorrow is "Children's Day." The best present I can get is not a toy but a promise that you will try to stop smoking.

I love you, Father.

(Signed by the child)

"Thus," Liu Baoyi continued, "the school curriculum and all the media events will point to the importance of No-Tobacco Day and Children's Day. We will work with local political leaders to promote the adoption of no-smoking policies in schools, other public buildings, and voluntarily in businesses. The local volunteer cancer organization will be making it known to everyone that free smoking-cessation clinics, at convenient hours, will be available for the entire month of June."

The National Chronic Disease Prevention Meeting was held in Tianjin, about 50 kilometers north of Beijing. Dr. Yu sat in the back of the auditorium. Although his demeanor was reserved on the outside, he was beaming on the inside as Shao Fang came to her closing remarks:

Again, there were 10,500 students (in grades two through six) in the intervention group and 9,987 students in the reference group. Although the knowledge scores were similar for the two groups at baseline, students in the intervention group had significantly higher knowledge scores (40 percent) at follow-up.

Smoking rates of fathers in both groups were the same at baseline (68 percent); that translated into 6,843 smokers in the intervention population. The stages-of-change data were also approximately the same—at baseline, 74 percent of smokers in the intervention group were precontemplatives, and the figure was 76 percent for smokers in the reference population. At follow-up, 61 percent of the precontemplatives in the intervention group reported a shift in stage to 'contemplation' or 'ready for action'; there was no significant shift among fathers in the reference group.

Finally, the data on smoking cessation were most encouraging. Self-reported data indicated that 90 percent of the 6,843 had quit for 10 days, 64 percent were still not smoking at 20 days, 30 percent by 60 days, and 11 percent by 210 days. For men in the reference population, only 2 percent reported a quit attempt in the first 10 days, and after 210 days the overall quit rate was 0.2 percent.

These findings suggest to us that a carefully planned, comprehensive tobacco-use prevention program that uses a school-based focus can be effective not only in improving the health knowledge of children, but also in predisposing previously unmotivated adults to quit smoking or at least to be more amenable to trying, and encouraging other adults who were somewhat motivated to actually try to quit.

Let me close with this epidemiological extrapolation: There are currently about 250 million smokers in China. If our program were implemented throughout the country and similar outcomes were attained, the result would be that 27 million smokers would have quit for 210 days. That is a dream we would very much like to pursue. Thank you.

The old horse smiled.

Case Analysis

The success of Li Fang's smoking-control efforts in China illustrates how a practitioner's understanding of theory can be directly applied to influence a health promotion program. We know that her thoughts about intervention were filtered through the lens of Stages of Change theory, and that those thoughts were influential in shaping the program that eventually emerged. We suspect that the thought processes of Li Fang and her co-workers probably went something like this:

Question: What portion of smokers are in the precomtemplative stage?

Action: Add Stages of Change questions to our baseline survey.

Answer: Our survey data tell us that a great majority of those who smoke are in the precontemplative stage.

Question: What does that tell us?

Answer: Three ideas stand out: (1) if we use methods aimed at smokers that emphasize the health hazards of smoking, or that implore smokers to join cessation clinics, such methods won't have much of an effect on smokers who are precontemplative; (2) it would be unrealistic for us to set quitting as the immediate goal; and (3) precontemplatives are resistant to cognitive messages that emphasize the detrimental health effects of tobacco; they are more likely to respond to *affective* approaches that appeal to more ultimate values than the value they hold for their own immediate health.

Actions: Our health problem is clear: tobacco causes unnecessary death and disability. Our program goal is also clear: to improve health by reducing the consumption of tobacco. Theory suggests that since behavior changes in stages, a prudent and scientifically sound first step would be to design and employ tactics that have a high probability of enhancing smokers' readiness to quit. One approach might be to try to move smokers from the precontemplation stage to the contemplation stage by appealing to a traditional Chinese value: Since elders hold a position of respect and honor in Chinese culture, it is their duty to pass their wisdom on to children. A possible message from children to their fathers might be, "Please don't do something that might compromise your ability to give me your wisdom and direction in the future."

From the perspective of health promotion practice, using theory is a lot like using a road map. First, you have to have a good idea about where you're going. Just as road maps can't help you if you don't know where you are going, theories have little practical value if you don't have a good grasp of the problem or issue you are trying to resolve. Most of the theories applied in health promotion programs are useful because they map out the process of how individuals, organizations, and communities change.

By understanding these processes, you can determine which roads are most likely to lead you to the outcomes you are seeking to achieve. Without a road map, you will be forced to do a lot of guessing about which road to take, which is likely to use up precious time and fuel. Similarly, inefficiency results when you try to frame interventions without applying theory. Thus, using theories to guide interventions will increase your chances of meeting program objectives and doing so in the most efficient way possible.

The remainder of this chapter is divided into two sections. The first provides an introductory discussion of theory, including a few ideas to help practitioners in the process of deciding what theories are most applicable to the specific circumstances they face. In the second section, we review several theories that are commonly applied by practitioners and provide examples of how elements of those theories inform the decisions practitioners make about interventions.

THEORY: A PRIMER

Consider this definition of theory: "a set of interrelated concepts, definitions, and propositions that present a *systematic* view of events or situations by specifying relationships among variables to *explain* or *predict* the events or situations."[3] [Italics added.] Whew! How does this academic definition translate into everyday actions?

Whether in our routine day-to-day tasks or our professional lives, our every action is grounded in some sort of "theory." In fact, we are hard-pressed to think of any conscious actions you might take *in absence of* some theory!

For example, consider the routine that many of us follow when arriving home after dark. We open the door, reach inside, and flip the light switch with the expectation that the lights will turn on. Whether consciously or not, our expectation is grounded in our belief that when we flip the switch, sufficient electrical current will flow to the light bulb socket and, assuming the light bulb is functional and properly affixed to the socket, the lights will go on.

Borrowing from the terms used in the definition cited previously, we put together *a set of interrelated concepts . . . and propositions* (switches, electrical current, light bulbs) which in turn give us a *systematic view of events* that help *specify relationships among variables.* (Flipping the switch activates electrical current and a causal chain of events, assuming that all parts of the system are functional.) These thought processes serve as the basis for *predicting an event* (the lights will go on!). Of course, most of us only become cognizant that we hold a "theory of house lighting" when we flip the switch and nothing happens. The dispatch and accompanying level of frustration we experience will in large part be determined by the steps we take to solve that problem—those with a faulty theory are likely to take more time and experience more frustration than those who act on a sound theory.

Activists and scholars from Saul Alinski and Paulo Freire to Meredith Minkler have consistently reminded practitioners to pay attention to the principle of participation and the process of respectfully engaging the community.[4] In Chapter 4 we discussed these important concepts not as theories per se but, as the title of this book implies, critical community health promotion ideas that work. As you proceed with the remainder of this chapter, you will note that it emphasizes theories that explain behavior and the precursors to behavior. Accordingly, we urge you to carefully examine this sampling of theories within the context of the community settings where they are inevitably played out.

Once the focus of the health promotion program (that is, the behavioral or environmental problem and the demographic, social, and economic context of that problem) has been clearly defined and agreed upon, practitioners may find it helpful to seek insights by finding the answers to three simple questions:

1. Is the theory relevant to my problem?

2. How does the theory help me understand targets for change?

3. How does the theory help in the selection or development of an intervention method or tactic?

Is the Theory Relevant to My Problem?

With detailed information about the kinds of behavioral and environmental factors that contribute to the problem, you can determine which theories, if any, provide a good explanation or understanding of the problem you've selected. For example, are those affected by the problem aware of the problem? Do they think it is a risk for them? Do they have the skills and motivation to take preventive action? Are solutions to the problem affordable and accessible? What kind of social pressures or social support would they experience for or against action? Depending upon the nature of the problem, some theories may be more useful than others. For many problems, especially complex ones, no single theory will fully address the problem, and it will be necessary to consider and combine multiple theories or parts of multiple theories.

How Does the Theory Help Me Understand Targets for Change?

Most theories propose a set of conditions or relationships under which changes are most likely to occur. In doing so, they implicitly identify targets for change. For example, if having a strong social support system is one of the key concepts in a particular theory of behavior change, that theory might predict that people with less social support would be less likely to make behavioral changes. Social support, then, is identified as one possible target for change. It follows that for this particular theory, effective programs designed to enhance social support should increase the likelihood of achieving the desired outcome.

How Does the Theory Help in the Selection or Development of an Intervention Method or Tactic?

Having identified from theories those concepts that are the best targets for health promotion programs, specific strategies must be developed to address those targets. Some theories go beyond explaining behavior, suggesting types of support or intervention to achieve or increase the likelihood of change. As in the previous example, if lack of social support was the cause of the problem, it follows from theory or theories that we would need to find ways to enhance social support. While there are many ways this can be done (*e.g.*, working with other family members, setting up a support group or telephone hotline, establishing an on-line computer user group), the challenge is selecting those tactics that will best address the problem as it exists in the population of interest. Unfortunately, there are no quick and easy ways to do this. Reading journal articles about other programs that have addressed the same problem can help you generate ideas, as can conversations with other practitioners and community members. Most important, whatever tactics you decide are best should be pretested with the members of the target population. Their evaluation of the appropriateness and usefulness of a program is critical.

THEORY SUMMARIES

Keeping in mind the spirit of the three questions discussed in the previous section, we will now describe and discuss four theories: the Health Belief Model, Self-Efficacy, the Theory of Reasoned Action, and Diffusion of Innovations Theory.[5] We highlight these theories because they contain the models most frequently applied by health promotion practitioners as a means to uncover clues that will lead them to the intervention approaches that best fit the problem and circumstances they face. They also fit variously with the predisposing, enabling, and reinforcing factors outlined in the previous chapters as part of the Precede/Proceed framework for planning. In presenting each theory, we will describe a particular health problem ("The Problem"), discuss what the theory says about behavior change in general and about this problem in particular ("The Theory"), and describe the intervention strategies suggested by the theory for addressing this problem ("The Solution").

The Health Belief Model

The Problem

Don Weiss is a pediatrician at an urban public health center in St. Louis, Missouri. The center's annual needs assessment showed that immunization rates among children age two years and younger were very low—fewer than half were fully immunized. Don knew something had to be done, but he wasn't sure what. At the next staff meeting, he asked several staff members to work with him in addressing the problem. He told them, "We've got to know why parents aren't bringing their kids in for shots. If we know the reasons, we can try to do something about it."

For several weeks, Don and his staff made it a point to interview personally all new parents who came in to the center for any reason. They also interviewed by telephone a number of the center's patients who had children age two and younger. They wanted to know what factors influenced parents' decisions to have their children immunized. When Don and his colleagues compared their notes after the next staff meeting, several clear patterns emerged:

- Parents did not know when and how many shots were recommended.
- Parents said their children looked healthy, and therefore must not need shots.
- Parents believed that childhood diseases were just a part of growing up, and not anything serious.
- Working parents could not get to the health center during its hours of operation.

- There were few public transportation routes to the health center.
- Compared to other demands and concerns, immunization just wasn't a high priority.

The Theory

The Health Belief Model (HBM) suggests that unless a person sees some value in making a behavior change, there will be no reason for him or her even to consider the change.[6] There are four main variables in the HBM—perceived susceptibility, perceived severity, perceived barriers, and perceived benefits. In short, the HBM suggests that behavior change is most likely to occur when a person believes he or she is at risk for a particular disease or health problem (perceived susceptibility), believes the consequences of getting that disease would be serious for him or her (perceived severity), and believes there are more benefits to be gained from changing the behavior (perceived benefits) than there are problems to overcome in changing the behavior (perceived barriers).

For Don Weiss and the problem of childhood immunization, the Health Belief model seemed to be a good fit. Many parents thought their babies didn't need shots (low perceived susceptibility) and thought that getting an immunizable childhood disease (*e.g.,* measles or mumps) was no big deal (low perceived severity). The center's hours weren't convenient for many parents, and public transportation to the clinic was limited (perceived barriers).

The Solution

According to the HBM, any program Don Weiss and his staff develop to promote childhood immunization should incorporate the following tactics:

- **Increase perceived susceptibility.** Help parents realize that their children may be at risk for preventable childhood diseases, even if they seem healthy.
- **Increase perceived severity.** Help parents understand that childhood diseases can be very serious and sometimes fatal.
- **Remove perceived barriers (or reduce perception of barriers as insurmountable).** Adopt evening and/or weekend hours to accommodate working parents; work with the public transportation authority to increase service to the health center.
- **Add perceived benefits (or increase the perception of the actual benefits).** Provide an incentive or reward to parents for their efforts in bringing their children to be immunized; help parents recognize how immunizations protect their children.

Note that if Don Weiss and his staff develop an immunization promotion program that addresses only some of these problems, it may be ineffective. For example, a program that increases the center's hours of operation without changing parents' beliefs that immunizations aren't important would have a limited impact. Yes, immunizations would be more accessible, but if parents didn't think they were important, their use would remain low. Note that the beliefs associated with these four dimensions of the model constitute predisposing factors in the Precede/Proceed model. It is possible sometimes to alter beliefs about environmental barriers and benefits without actually changing the environment, enabling factors, or reinforcing factors. It is also possible to change the beliefs or perceptions of barriers and benefits by directly changing the enabling and reinforcing factors.

Self-Efficacy

The Problem

Janis Whitlock is the director of the student health center at a large midwestern university. In addition to providing primary-care services for students, the center offers a variety of educational programs, peer counseling, and an orientation for all incoming freshmen. In the past, Janis and her staff had developed innovative programs to prevent alcohol-related injuries and date rape. Now they had a new challenge. For the third year in a row, the rate of sexually transmitted diseases among students reporting symptoms at the student health service has increased. Promoting safe sex practices on campus had always been one of Janis's top priorities, but she knew the center was going to have to do a better job.

With the help of two health education faculty members from the School of Health Sciences, Janis developed a survey to assess students' beliefs and practices about sexual activity and their use of the center's programs. Janis told the faculty members, "Either our programs aren't addressing the real problem, they aren't reaching the students, or both. We need to know where to direct our energy." The anonymous survey was mailed to a random sample of 800 undergraduate students, of whom 468 responded. The survey showed the following results among sexually active students:

- Only 16 percent said they use a condom every time they have sex.
- Only 26 percent had ever initiated a discussion about condom use with a sex partner.
- 79 percent, including 92 percent of females, said that they could not easily discuss condom use with a sex partner.
- 66 percent, including 75 percent of females, said that talking about condom use with a sex partner probably would not make condom use any more acceptable.
- 43 percent of females said that it was likely that asking a sex partner to use a condom would make the partner angry.

The Theory

Self-Efficacy is really not a theory itself, but rather an important concept in Bandura's social learning theory.[7] According to social learning theory, individuals who believe they are capable of taking some specific action and who believe that taking that action will lead to a desirable outcome are most likely to change. A person's beliefs about his or her ability to make a particular change are called *efficacy expectations* or *self-efficacy*. Beliefs about whether making that change will lead to a particular outcome are called *outcome expectations*. Both beliefs work together to affect a person's actions. For example, if a person believes that she can make a change, but sees no value resulting from her efforts, the chances of her taking action are slim. Likewise, if she believes that making the change would be valuable for her, but does not feel she is capable of making the change, it is unlikely to occur. It is important to note that beliefs about self-efficacy are always specific to some action, not a personality trait. For example, a person may have very high self-efficacy beliefs for changing one behavior, but low self-efficacy beliefs for changing another.

The results from the student survey suggest that the concepts of self-efficacy and outcome expectations may help explain the high rate of sexually transmitted diseases Janis's health center has observed. For sexually active persons, consistent condom use is necessary to prevent the spread of STDs. But as the survey showed, few students use condoms regularly. Why not? The data shown earlier suggest that many students felt that they weren't able to talk to a partner about condom use (low self-efficacy). Furthermore, many believed that talking to a partner about condom use wouldn't make using condoms any more acceptable, and might even anger some partners (negative outcome expectations). Given these survey results, social learning theory would predict that condom use would be low in this population, and therefore STD rates could be high.

The Solution

There are four main factors that affect self-efficacy—*personal experience, observational experience, verbal persuasion,* and *physiological state*. For example, a student may have high self-efficacy for starting a conversation about condom use because she had done it before (personal experience), because she had attended a class where videotapes and role plays showed other people starting such a conversation (observational experience), because she had been reassured by friends that she could do it (verbal persuasion), or because she didn't get nervous and feel sick when she thought about doing it (no physiological arousal).

Thus, social learning theory would suggest that a program designed to enhance low self-efficacy for negotiating condom use with a sex partner might include some of the following intervention strategies:

- **Teach and model specific behavioral and communication skills for negotiating condom use.** Seeing others demonstrate these skills will help students learn and adopt them.
- **Provide opportunities for students to rehearse these behavioral and communication skills.** Practicing, even in simulations, is valuable experience.
- **Make the initial objectives of the program relatively simple for students to achieve.** For example, an objective might be to ask your partner any one question about condoms the next time you are together. Successes, no matter how small, can help build self-efficacy for future actions. Participants also need to rehearse how to handle this one question because failure, no matter how small, can sometimes discourage them from proceeding to the next step.
- **Focus on the positive aspects of an incomplete performance.** Even in an unsuccessful attempt to initiate discussion about condom use, the student should be able to focus on something positive. Finding and emphasizing that something can offset damage to self-efficacy.
- **Provide reinforcement and encouragement.** Hearing that others believe in you, or think you can do it, builds self-efficacy.
- **Teach relaxation skills.** Students who feel very nervous, become short of breath, or perspire when thinking about talking to a partner about condom use may interpret these signs as meaning they won't be able to do it. Knowing how to calm yourself down can help prevent losing self-efficacy.

To help change negative outcome expectations, a program should clearly demonstrate the relationship between the behavior of interest and the outcome. Where possible, it should provide opportunities for students to experience specific outcomes that may result from the actions they have (or have not) taken. In designing exercises that do this, it may be especially important to think about the outcomes of a behavior as immediate and tangible, not as long-term health risks or benefits.

Again, self-efficacy fits within the predisposing factors of the Precede/Proceed model, but it can be related to other aspects of Social Learning Theory that fit more clearly under enabling and reinforcing factors.

The Theory of Reasoned Action

The Problem

Lincoln Phillips is a graduate student getting a master's degree in public health. For his thesis project, he is working with Forever Yours Senior Center, a large organization that offers programs to over 2,000 senior residents in the Lakewood area adjacent to the university. Lincoln's primary interest is to develop and implement physical activity programs for older adults. Lincoln had seen his grandmother suffer the consequences of osteoporosis, had read about the low rates of physical activity in aging populations, and thought this was an area of real need where he could make a difference. As he'd learned in his classes, his first step was to conduct a needs assessment. He spent weeks talking with staff members from agencies and organizations that served older adults, with family members of older adults, and with older adults themselves at the Forever Yours center, in coffee shops and in their homes. As he completed more and more interviews, he could see several clear patterns emerging:

- Most older adults believed that, at their age, there was little benefit from physical activity.
- Many older adults reported that their friends and neighbors were not physically active.
- Many older adults and some family members thought of physical activity as jogging or bicycling, as they saw the "young people" in the park doing.
- Many family members of older adults thought physical activity would be dangerous for their relatives.

The Theory

According to the Theory of Reasoned Action, the best predictor of a person taking some health-related action is whether the person *intends* to take action.[8] The theory specifies that a person's intention is determined by two factors—the person's attitude toward the behavior, and what the person thinks other people would want him or her to do regarding the behavior. A person's attitudes are made up of:

- beliefs about outcomes that may result from engaging in the behavior, and
- beliefs about how desirable or undesirable those outcomes are.

A person's perceptions of others' beliefs are determined by:

- what the person thinks others would like him or her to do regarding the behavior, and
- how much or little the person wants to comply with what others think he or she should do.

In summary, when a person believes a behavior will lead to some valuable outcome, and believes that others whom that person respects and wants to please think he or she should engage in the behavior, then the person is more likely to *intend* to take action, and therefore is more likely to act.

Lincoln remembered the Theory of Reasoned Action from his classes on behavior change theory and saw that it really applied to his project with the senior center. Many of the older adults he talked to saw little benefit to be gained from doing physical activity, and some even thought it could hurt them. Clearly they had a negative attitude toward physical activity. In addition, few of their friends and neighbors were physically active, and some members of their families thought exercising could be risky for them. If the older adults valued or respected the opinions of their friends and family members, this too would undermine any attempt he made to promote physical activity with this population.

The Solution

Lincoln realized that among other things, the program he developed would need to address older adults' negative attitudes about physical activity, and their perceptions of how the important people in their lives felt about them doing physical activity. Reviewing the Theory of Reasoned Action, he saw several possible solutions. To change older adults' attitudes about physical activity, he could:

- **Add a new, positive belief.** "Physical activity like walking is safe and beneficial, can be a social activity with friends, and can reduce your risk of injury by making your body stronger."
- **Reinforce an existing positive belief.** "Remember how much you used to enjoy a more active lifestyle? Regular physical activity can help you become that way again."
- **Challenge an existing negative belief.** "You think you're too old to exercise, but doctors and other health experts say it's one of the best things you can do for yourself no matter what your age."
- **Enhance the perceived desirability of a new or existing belief.** "The stronger you are, the less you'll have to rely on others, the longer you'll be able to live independently, and the more you can play with your grandchildren."

To change older adults' beliefs about what others want them to do, he could:

- **Change the attitudes of the important others.** Help family members and friends recognize the value of physical activity for older adults, and ask them to support and encourage their efforts to be more active.
- **Add new "others" to their lives.** Introduce new social contacts, such as members of a mall walking club, a doctor, or a pharmacist, who support physical activity.
- **Challenge their beliefs about what others think they should do.** "Actually, your friends, your family, and your doctor all think it would

be a *good* idea for you to become more active—why don't you ask them?"

- **Change the motivation to comply with others.** "You shouldn't be so concerned about what Mr. Jones thinks; your doctor and your family think it's a good idea for you to be physically active."

Diffusion of Innovations Theory

The Problem

One month later, Lincoln had developed a comprehensive physical activity program for the Forever Yours Senior Center based in combination on (1) the insight he gained on the attitudes of seniors by using the Theory of Reasoned Action, and (2) intervention ideas he received as a result of correspondence with Drs. Michael Pratt and Carl Casperson, physical activity experts at the CDCP. Lincoln shared his proposed program with his faculty advisor, who concurred that his use of the Theory of Reasoned Action was indeed appropriate, and then added, "Is there anything else you might do to maximize the chance that the seniors will actually undertake the activities you are now prepared to offer?"

As Lincoln prepared his response, the professor said, "Take another look at Diffusion of Innovations Theory and see if any ideas crop up."

The Theory

Diffusion of Innovations Theory has its origins in communications and, interestingly, agriculture.[9] It explains how, over time, a new idea or product (an innovation) gains momentum and spreads (diffuses) through a given population. *Adoption* is a key word in the context of this theory—simply translated, it means to do something (*e.g.,* think, believe, purchase, act, or behave) in a way that you haven't previously. Thus, new ideas and products spread in a population or society to the extent that people "adopt" them. The notion of an adoption spreading through a population implies of course, that not everyone jumps on the bandwagon immediately. Some do; but others are more conservative and wait it out, perhaps looking for evidence that the innovation in question is not just a passing fancy.

Researchers have noted that those who adopt an innovation early in the diffusion process seem to demonstrate characteristics that are different from those who adopt with the majority, and differ still more from those who adopt later. Those who are the first to take up a new idea, product, or action are called innovators; they are followed, in order, by early adopters, the early majority, the later majority, and finally the late adopters (sometimes unkindly labeled *laggards*). Generally, simple exposure to and a reasonable level of comprehension of the innovation is sufficient to trigger adoption by innovators. The level of effort required to predict adoption becomes incrementally greater for those in the early-adopter, early-majority, and later-majority groups.

Examples of adopting an innovation within the commercial sector include purchasing a color TV in 1970, a CD player in 1980, and a cellular phone in 1990. Examples in the health sector would include seeking out influenza vaccinations in 1970, purchasing and drinking skim milk in 1980, and passing indoor clean air policies and tobacco excise tax legislation in 1990.

As you will note in the examples given, some adoption decisions have impact beyond the individual level. As Glanz and Rimer so correctly point out, when teachers adopt a new school health curriculum, when a worksite manager contracts for new screening services, and when a city council adopts a recycling policy, the impact obviously extends far beyond the individual.[10]

An important aspect of this theory for practitioners is that five characteristics about the innovation itself appear to have a strong influence on the extent to which the product or recommended action will be adopted. Table 5.1 provides a definition of each of the characteristics and an explanation of how, if unattended, each characteristic could inhibit adoption.

Practitioners who understand the theory of adoption routinely test their program ideas against these characteristics—a brilliant, scientifically and theoretically sound idea won't be used if the intended users see it as too complicated and potentially at odds with their values. For example, the Washington Heights–Inwood Heart Health Program is a community-based heart disease prevention program serving a low-income community population of 240,000 people in inner-city New York. In reporting their six-year evaluation results, researchers described a comprehensive "low-fat milk campaign" (involving school, community, and policy components) that was remarkably successful in lowering the intake of saturated fat among children in the community. In describing the factors contributing to the success of the intervention, the investigators said:

> The recommended behavioral change was easy to understand and simple to do, did not impose time commitments or significant monetary costs, was readily accepted by children, involved fun and interactive campaign activities, and emphasized positive messages and social reinforcements in campaign themes. (Shea, Basch, Wechsler, Lantiqua, p.167)[11]

The Solution

Lincoln asked for and received permission from the Forever Yours Senior Center director to make arrangements to meet with several groups of senior participants. He scheduled three small group sessions of about ten seniors

TABLE 5-1   Diffusion of Innovations Theory

Concept	Definition	Reasons for Not Adopting
Relative advantage	The degree to which an innovation is seen as better than the idea, practice, program, or product it replaces	Benefits not evident: *e.g.,* no apparent savings, doesn't give me more than I have, doesn't save time
Compatibility	How consistent the innovation is with values, habits, experience, and needs of potential adopters	Not consistent with my values: *e.g.,* I believe in the right to bear arms and your policy restricts my ability to buy guns
Complexity	How difficult the innovation is to understand and/or use	Too complicated: *e.g.,* I can't do your weight-loss program because it means I have to get a babysitter
Trialability	The extent to which the innovation can be experimented with before a commitment to adopt is required	You won't let me see if I like it, so no thanks; will you guarantee it?
Observability	The extent to which the innovation provides tangible or visible results	How do I know it will work; I don't see anyone else doing it

per group. In leisurely settings that included coffee, tea, and cookies, Lincoln carried on a discussion with each group that lasted about an hour or so. After appropriate introductions, he described the activities that were likely to be included in the program and then structured the discussions so that he could get a sense of the seniors' reactions based on the five concepts described in Table 5.1.

Relative Advantage.   He discovered that some of the seniors wondered whether the effort was really "worth it." As Lincoln briefly described some of the benefits of physical activity to the seniors, he noted that a rather large number of them were unaware of the fact that exercising had direct benefits for them "even at this late stage." As a result, he thought of several possible tactics:

1. Have a doctor and/or physical therapist visit with the seniors and their families to discuss the numerous benefits of exercise to this age group; for example, many conditions can be prevented or their symptoms reduced

by appropriate exercise (thereby resulting in fewer visits to the doctor and less frequent hospitalization), and physiological changes resulting from exercise can increase feelings of physical and mental well-being (thereby improving mood and relieving symptoms of depression). The speaker could reassure the audience about the safety of exercise and suggest that those who have specific health concerns could have a simple and routine medical check with their doctor before the programs commence.

2. Have a social worker or member of the clergy talk to the FYSC about the benefits of the social aspects of exercise, including friendship, team building, and the enrichment of community life.

3. Assistance from the "opinion leaders" in the FYSC can be enlisted to maximize members' attendance at these presentations, and later to generate discussion and active participation in aspects of program implementation. This can be achieved through informal channels using established social networks within the FYSC. The higher the level of members' early involvement in priority setting and suggesting how the programs might best be run, the higher the participation rates will be.

Compatibility.   Lincoln found that seniors wanted the activity program to "fit in" with their lifestyles, interests, and abilities. Some of the activities could encompass or expand upon things that the seniors were already doing in their daily lives (for example, walking to shops instead of taking the bus).

He also found out that the social aspects were very important. Therefore, it would be useful to incorporate an opportunity for socializing, perhaps over tea or coffee, after some of the activities—some people implied that such social contact was more attractive to them than the physical activity.

This insight triggered the following ideas:

1. Offer a variety of programs, as people differ widely in the types of exercise that appeal to them. Activities such as dancing and cycling, for example, may have particular appeal to many seniors because they may well have had good experiences with these in their younger days or view them as truly recreational. Other factors necessitating a variety of programs are the weather, as certain activities may be impractical or lack appeal on cool or wet days, and the fact that some activities may be unsuitable for people with particular medical conditions. Options might include:

   • graded walks in groups, where the exercise is combined with social interaction

   • ballroom or "old-time" dancing evenings

   • exercise classes such as "Fun and Fitness for the Over 60s", including (stationary) exercise bicycles and a variety of other exercises

   • swimming

2. Regularly consult members to determine which types of activity are of interest, and ask the "opinion leaders" to encourage suggestions and discussion on the issues involved.

Complexity.   Most participants did not find Lincoln's proposed activities to be at all too complex. However, they did express concern about their friends whose mobility was seriously impaired and who were restricted to wheelchairs or walkers. What could be done to make activities amenable to them as well? As he thought about this concern, no good ideas came to Lincoln's mind. The fact was, he knew little about physical activity for senior citizens who were handicapped. He made a mental note to consult with his professor and also a friend who was a physical therapy student.

Trialability.   In each of the three discussion groups, at least one or two people had expressed the desire to "test the waters" with the activities, without pressure or obligation and before any commitment to sign up was required. Several thoughts came to Lincoln's mind:

- Offer participation in the activity for an initial trial period, making it clear that there is no obligation to continue taking part afterward.
- Provide an incentive to come to the first session (*e.g.,* discounts at the local sports clothing retailer, grocery store, or pharmacy).
- Provide home pickups and return transportation.

Observability.   During the discussions, participants raised three questions: (1) Were they the first ones to try this kind of activity? (2) Were there really visible benefits from the innovations Lincoln was proposing? and (3) Were they more likely to participate in them? Lincoln thought of several ways he might address these questions:

- Enlist the help of members of the FYSC or members of the public who have reaped the benefits of exercise, and who are willing to give short talks to members about how it has changed their lives in measurable ways (*e.g.,* weight loss, reduced blood pressure, increased stamina, more mobility resulting in fewer arthritic symptoms). Appropriate photographs or slides of "before and after" may be useful in illustrating these messages.
- Later, when programs have been running for some time, recruit "innovators" and "early adopters" to give these talks, and to discuss and demonstrate their successes in less formal settings within the FYSC social networks, in order to increase program participation rates.
- When promoting or advertising the programs, display photographs on the bulletins of groups of seniors taking part in the activities (from other centers, towns, states, etc.) to demonstrate that other seniors' groups already run these programs and find them enjoyable. For exam-

ple, photographs of happy groups at a social dance, or groups of seniors walking and talking in a shady park, could appeal to many people and induce them to join up.

• In order to be able to quantify the benefits of exercise, it is useful to encourage participants to keep a simple record of some measurements over time (*e.g.,* weight, distance walked with ease, time taken to swim a certain distance). These records help to demonstrate objectively the improvements gained by program participation and can be used to encourage others to take part.

SUMMARY

We have all heard Kurt Lewin's oft-cited aphorism that there is nothing so practical as a good theory. This leads us to make at least two assumptions: (1) "good theories" exist, and (2) those theories are sufficiently well understood to be put to use.

In practical terms, theories are "good" to the extent that they help us understand how things work. There is ample empirical research indicating that theories give us clues, some of which are highly predictive, of the key factors, forces, and conditions that influence health status and health behaviors. Our counsel to practitioners is to become familiar with those theories and their elements and continually use that knowledge to probe for the little insights could make big differences in the effects of a health promotion program. Shao Fang was using such a probe when her new understanding of Stages of Change Theory prompted her to wonder: "If a large number of men in the Eastern District are not in the ready for action stage, a large campaign on smoking cessation may not be a good investment of time and effort." For Shao Fang, a good theory was indeed practical.

As more research in community health promotion is undertaken, more theories will come to light. As long as health promotion practitioners view theories as useful and practical tools, they will be readily incorporated into more robust and effective programs. In the next Chapter on Tactics, notice how the application of theory influences decisions regarding intervention strategies and tactics.

ENDNOTES

1. By using the example of Stages of Change Theory, we are not saying that it is the best or even the most appropriate theory to use in Li Fang's case. We use this example to illustrate how a working knowledge of theory can influence decisions made when one is planning an outcome-oriented health promotion program. As our awareness of various theories expands, so too does our profes-

sional responsibility to justify our preference of one theory over another or to combine the most relevant elements of several theories. For added information on Stages of Change Theories, we suggest the writing of James Prochaska, beginning with: Prochaska JO, DiClemente CC, Norcross JC. In search of how people change: applications to addictive behaviors. *Am Psychologist.* 1992;47: 1102–1114.

2. World No-Tobacco Day is an annual event that encourages governments, communities, and other groups to become aware of the hazards of tobacco and encourages those who use tobacco to quit for at least one day. Children's Day is a Chinese holiday celebrating the importance of nurturing children.

3. Glanz K, Rimer BK. *Theory at a Glance: A Guide for Health Promotion Practice.* Washington, DC: U.S. Department of Health and Human Services, National Institutes of Health; 1986:11.

4. For basic readings in the fundamental principles of community organization and participation, we recommend: Alinski SD. *Reveille for Radicals.* Chicago: University of Chicago; 1969; and Freire P. *Education for Critical Consciousness.* New York: Sebury Press; 1973. For direct health promotion applications of those principles we suggest: Minkler, M. Improving health through community organization. In: Glanz K, Marcus-Lewis F, Rimer B, eds. *Health Behavior and Education: Theory, Research and Practice.* San Francisco: Jossey-Bass; 1990.

5. The Transtheoretical Model, or Stages of Change Theory, is a frequently applied thesis in health promotion. It is not included here because it is a component in the Old Horse case story.

6. For background reading on the Health Belief Model, we suggest: Becker MH ed. The health belief model and personal health behavior. *Health Education Monographs.* 1974;2:324–473; Rosenstock IM. Historical origins of the health belief model. *Health Education Monographs.* 1974;2:470–473; Janz NK, Becker MH. The health belief model: a decade later. *Health Educ Q.* 1984;11:1–47; and Becker MH, Haefner D, Kasl SV, et al. Selected psychosocial models and correlates of individual health-related behaviors. *Med Care.* 1977; 15(suppl):27–46.

7. For background reading on Social Learning Theory, we suggest: Bandura A. Toward a unifying theory of behavior change. *Psychological Review.* 1977;84(2):191–215; Bandura A. *Social Foundations of Thought and Action.* Englewood Cliffs, NJ: Prentice-Hall; 1986; and Strecker VJ, DeVillis BM, Becker MH, Rosenstock IM. The role of self efficacy in achieving health behavior change. *Health Educ Q.* 1986;13:73–92.

8. For further reading on the Theory of Reasoned Action, we suggest: Ajzen I, Fishbein M. *Understanding Attitudes and Predicting Social Behavior.* Englewood Cliffs, NJ: Prentice-Hall; 1980; and Jorgenson SR, Sonstegard JS. Predicting adolescent sexual and contraceptive behavior: an application and test to the Fishbein model. *J Marriage Family.* 1984;46:43–55.

9. For further reading on Diffusion of Innovations Theory, we suggest: Rogers EM, *The Diffusion of Innovations.* 3rd ed. New York: Free Press; 1983; Basch CD, Eveland JD, Portnoy B. Diffusion systems for education and learning about health, *Family and Community Health.* 1986;9:1–26; and Orlandi MA. The diffusion and adoption of worksite health promotion innovations: an analysis of barriers. *Preventive Medicine.* 1987;16:119–130.

10. Glanz K, Rimer BK. *Theory at a Glance: A Guide for Health Promotion Practice.* Washington, DC: U.S. Department of Health and Human Services, National Institutes of Health, 1986.
11. Shea S, Basch C, Wechsler H, Lantiqua R. The Washington Heights–Inwood healthy heart program: a 6-year report from a disadvantaged urban setting, *AJPH.* 1996;86(2):166–171.

CHAPTER 6

Tactics

Home

Everyone in the family looked forward to the annual Thanksgiving gathering at the Rodriguez home in Salinas, California. Edgar and Carla Rodriguez had three children: two daughters, one son, and a ten-month old grandchild, Esther. This year's gathering was special because Edgar and Carla's son, Ray, was coming home from Germany for the first time in two years.

Outside the Rodriguez household, Ray was known as Captain Raymond E. Rodriguez, U.S. Air Force. Ray had gone to Fresno State University on a football scholarship but suffered a career-ending knee injury in his sophomore year. It was during his rehabilitation that he discovered his interest in the field of physical therapy. After graduating and completing his training as a certified physical therapist, he accepted a commission in the Air Force. Ray specialized in rehabilitating patients suffering from mission- and work-related injuries; in the process, he distinguished himself as a superb therapist and a first-rate administrator—he was a "people person." Nearly ten years of working on the restorative side of health in the Air Force had firmed up Ray's desire to become more involved in prevention.

One month before Thanksgiving, Ray received news that he had been selected to supervise an Air Force Health and Wellness Center (HAWC). Air Force policy calls for one of these centers to be established at every Air Force installation for the purpose of providing planned programs in health promotion and disease prevention for active-duty personnel, military retirees, their dependents, and civilian employees. It was the right job at the right time for Ray; he was assigned to Dobbins Air Force Base just outside Atlanta, Georgia.

During the Thanksgiving holiday, Ray rediscovered the reality of family life: tight sleeping quarters, chairs squeezed around the dinner table, lines for the bathroom, a few debates about who was going to be responsible for what, too much food, and a house full of people who couldn't care less about their wild-looking morning hair! He marveled at how five days of such joyful chaos relieved the tension in his body.

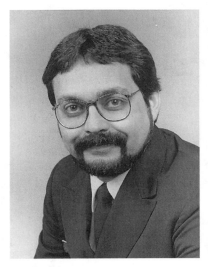

Ray Rodriguez

As always, the good-byes were tearful. Ray anticipated the stress that would be caused by hordes of travelers. After negotiating the holiday traffic on the two-hour drive from Salinas to San Francisco International Airport and enduring the usual scheduling delays, he finally settled in his seat for his flight to Atlanta.

*   *   *

Colonel Tim Gayle, chief of health promotion activities and programs for the entire U.S. Air Force, had sent Ray a packet of materials to review in preparation for a two-day seminar on health promotion for all HAWC directors in the southeastern region. Just after takeoff, Ray reached down for his briefcase under the seat in front of him, extracted a stack of articles, picked one out, and started to read, making occasional notes in the margins.

Although Ray was gregarious and made friends easily, he had learned that most travelers like the privacy of their space, so he had made it a habit not to initiate conversation on an airplane. But after a few minutes, the woman sitting next to him asked, "Excuse me, are you involved with health reform?"

Ray shrugged his shoulders, "Oh, well, not directly—why do you ask?"

"I couldn't help seeing the title of that article, 'Planning for Health Promotion,' and I just thought . . .'"

Ray politely interrupted with a chuckle, "Well, I am in the health field." He went on to explain that he was catching up on some reading for a briefing he was going to have about his new assignment at Dobbins Air Force Base. He stuck out his hand. "I'm Ray Rodriguez."

"Lela Davis. Nice to meet you, Ray."

"Are you in the health field as well?" Ray asked.

"No, I've been involved with city planning for over 10 years, the last five of which have been in Atlanta; actually, I'm a demographer by training!" Lela gestured to the flight attendant. "May I have a cup of coffee, please?"

"Cream and sugar?"

"Just cream, thank you," Lela said.

The flight attendant looked at Ray. "And you, sir?"

Ray held up the palm of his hand. "I'm fine, thanks."

Ray enjoyed the art of conversation. At that very moment, he would rather exchange thoughts with Lela than plow through his readings! In just a few minutes, it became clear that Ray and Lela shared a common interest in strategic planning. During the course of their casual conversation, Lela commented, "During the time I've worked on community planning, the most interesting and practical interpretation of strategic planning was given to me by a friend who is an accomplished chess player."

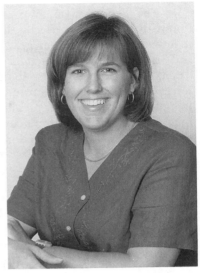

Lela Davis

"Not that guy who beat the computer?" Ray asked.

"Kasparov?" Lela chuckled. "No, not him. Do you play chess?"

"Used to," Ray said pensively, "but I haven't played in years." He thought of his early teen years in Salinas, when his father had taught him to play with a set of chess pieces carved out of shiny marble. But along with many other small pleasures, chess had given way to football.

Lela went on: "Anyway, here's what my chess player friend said: When accomplished players start the game, neither player is certain of the approach his or her opponent is going to take. So, in the beginning, the players are basically checking each other out—looking for possible openings and clues on what to do next. Their interpretation of these clues leads to the formulation of their overall plan or strategy. When they are confident of their strategic plan, it is simply a matter of applying the specific tactics most likely to lead to the capture of the queen."

Ray grinned and nodded. "So, in other words, strategic planning is what you do when you *don't* know what to do; tactics are what you do when you *know* what to do!"

Lela laughed. "Right on, Captain! But, as is usually the case, the devil is in the details."

"Meaning?" Ray asked.

Lela took a sip of her coffee. "Meaning that when you're dealing with the kind of planning that both of us do—involving people with differing beliefs, politics, and views—cookie-cutter approaches won't get the job done. You have to be flexible and strategic with your tactics. In the kind of community planning I do, I have found that even the most tried-and-true methods have to be adapted to the unique needs of a community or neighborhood." That made sense to Ray.

The flight to Atlanta was a smooth one. Ray reflected on his conversation with Lela—how perfectly the chess metaphor explained the process he followed as a physical therapist. First, a team of health workers diagnosed and assessed the extent of injury and trauma suffered by a given patient. Then, that information, combined with a detailed history of the patient, served as the basis for the formulation of an intervention plan. Ray's role in that plan was to choose or prescribe the combination of therapies most likely to yield the best health outcome based on the patient assessment. It was precisely that skill that helped give Ray his much-deserved reputation as a first-rate practitioner; he knew the importance of a good diagnosis and had the ability to strategically apply the combination of therapeutic tactics most likely to be effective.

Ray's thoughts shifted to his new situation. He was confident that he and his colleagues in the HAWC at Dobbins would be able to do the strategic planning part, but the tactical or application part of effective health promotion and disease prevention was another matter. Lela's chess story brought to light something Ray had perhaps unconsciously pushed into the shadows: Health promotion tactics or methods were something he needed to know much more about.

With that thought, Ray returned to his stack of readings. He finished the first article and turned to the next one, which had a handwritten note from Colonel Gayle stapled to the first page:

Ray:

Although this article is a few years old, I think it illustrates how multiple methods of health promotion can be applied to a single problem. I created a modification of the authors' table that we have used in some seminars and workshops—we have found the table a useful tool to help people see how the different attributes of various health promotion methods can be combined to create what we call a comprehensive approach. Hope it helps. See you in Atlanta.

Tim

Ray read the article. It had been published by Donald Reid and some of his fellow health promotion workers in England and described various intervention options that might be employed in a comprehensive tobacco-use prevention and control program at the national level.[1] The modified table that Colonel Gayle mentioned in his note was laid out in a matrix (Figure 6.1). The leftmost column provided a listing of general categories of intervention approaches, or tactics. Five other columns each represented a particular piece of information about each tactic. The cells of the matrix were empty. Colonel Gayle had attached a list of simple definitions, next to which he had written another note for Ray:

Problem: _____

Objective: _____

Tactic	Effectiveness	Reach	Acceptability	Cost	Public Support
Health Communications					
Media Advocacy					
Policy Actions					
School					
Workplace					
Health Care Setting					

FIGURE 6.1   Colonel Tim Gayle's Modification of the Reid et al. Table

Ray:

In our training, we ask participants to consider several types of intervention "tactics" (e.g., school health, mass media, policy development, etc.) and "evidence" that will enable them to put information in the open cells of the matrix. Then we have them talk with their fellow participants and come to a consensus as to what information should go into each cell.

Tim

The definitions for each of the criteria listed in the column headings were listed below the table:

- **Effectiveness**—the extent to which there is evidence that, when properly applied, this tactic will contribute to attaining the objective for which it was chosen.
- **Reach**—the potential for reaching a large proportion of the target audience.
- **Acceptability**—the extent to which the target audience, general public, and relevant agencies find the tactic to be within the range of actions that are socially and culturally acceptable.
- **Cost**—the extent to which the proper application of the tactic is economically feasible.
- **Public Support**—the extent to which the effective application of a tactic has potential for engendering positive public opinion and, therefore, support for either the issue in particular, or public health and prevention in general.

Ray thought to himself how the matrix reminded him of a chess board.

Case Analysis

We don't know whether Captain Rodriguez got off the airplane with more insight about the job he was about to undertake than he had when he boarded a few hours earlier. However, we do know that the chess analogy reminded him that an effective intervention requires two complementary skills, both of which must be applied strategically: (1) the ability to carry out a sound analysis of the health problem and the multiple factors associated with that problem, and (2) the knowledge and capacity to apply the methods or tactics most likely to effectively address that problem. The previous chapters in this book have attended primarily to issues related to the former set of skills; we now focus on the latter.

Over the years, we have had the pleasure of meeting and visiting with experienced health promotion practitioners from around the globe. In spite of language and cultural differences, we have observed that effective practitioners seem to act on a common set of ideas that work for them as they make decisions about selecting the tactics most likely to achieve their program objectives. We offer these ideas in hopes that they might stimulate the development of a mental model for those charged with the responsibility of implementing a community health promotion program.

Idea 1: Use Objectives to Stay Focused

Not only do effective practitioners take seriously the task of identifying practical, specific, and measurable objectives, but they revisit those objectives often to make sure they are on track.[2] Recall our earlier reference to the children's pedestrian-injury prevention project in Perth, Australia; project staff had affixed a flow chart of their program plan, including specific intervention objectives, on their office wall. They found this simple technique to be an effective means to help them keep their intervention ideas focused on program objectives. (See Tables 3.1 and 3.2.)

Idea 2: Make Informed Decisions

Simply put, the probability that you will select methods and tactics that will work (achieve your program objectives) increases proportionately with your understanding of the people and the environment where the intervention is to take place. All effective practitioners use some routine process to assess existing levels of knowledge, attitudes, capacities, and environmental supports. Their ultimate intervention decisions are shaped by their interpretation of the information they obtain from that process in light of behavioral, social, and learning theory.

Idea 3: Don't Reinvent the Wheel

Like accomplished athletes, experienced practitioners waste little "motion" because they know the wisdom of simplicity. For health promotion practitioners, simplicity begins with taking the time to see and confirm what the community already has to offer before trying to envision new intervention ideas. Often, fine-tuning a program already in place will suffice and is likely to have the added benefit of demonstrating respect for prior efforts undertaken by the community.

Idea 4: There Is No Such Thing as a Free Lunch

We all know of creative practitioners who have used volunteers or have been able to secure a *pro bono* component for a given aspect of a health promotion program. But one must take care not to mistake these creative actions with the reality that it takes economic and human resources to implement and sustain a program over time. For experienced practitioners, the decision to select a given intervention method or tactic will in part be determined by the estimated costs of implementing that method.

We have found it helpful to think of three categories of costs: economic costs, time costs, and opportunity costs. Economic costs include such things as salaries and benefits, materials, equipment, printing, and media time. Time is a cost in the sense that it is a necessary commodity for planning and preparation; when planners do not allow sufficient time for preparation and coordination among sectors, they put their programs at risk for failure. Finally, when colleagues agree to lend you their personal support for your program, that means they have to give up or lower their level of effort on something else; this is an opportunity cost. Recall the case story of Linda Thomas in Chapter 1. Even though she held the stress management sessions during her own lunch time, the project absorbed her attention, energy, and at least some portion of her time. Thus, her decision to devote time to the stress reduction effort did have a cost in that it diminished and took away from the opportunity to invest her energy in another program.

Idea 5: To Maximize Effectiveness, Strategically Combine Multiple Tactics to Influence Complex Problems

Matrices such as that one illustrated in the "Checkmate" case story give us the kind of information that helps ensure that all of the key issues are being addressed, that we are taking a strategic and comprehensive approach. After an exhaustive review of the most effective environmental and policy tactics to reduce tobacco use, Brownson and his colleagues provided this wisdom about the importance of comprehensiveness:[3]

> Environmental and policy interventions may have greater impact
> if they are carried out over multiple settings—health care, schools,
> or worksites, in addition to the whole community. (p. 480)

Idea 6: Monitor the Intervention Process and Make Changes as Needed

Generally, effective health promotion practitioners hold a subtle and practical view of evaluation. That is, they see evaluation not so much as a tool to prove that their programs are working, but more as a means to answer the question, "*How* is the program working?" For example, they look for information that will help them answer questions such as, "Are we following our intervention protocols correctly?" or, "Are we reaching the populations we have set out to reach?" They seek to find "bad" news as well as "good" news, because they understand that all programs will experience their share of problems, especially in the formative stages. One of the hallmarks of an effective program is that planners take creative corrective action triggered by the detection of "bad" news.

Idea 7: Use Science to Enhance Your Creativity

Media advocacy pioneer Mike Pertschuk once said this about his own specialty: "Media advocacy requires art, imagination, and creativity; any attempt to reduce it to a series of rigid and prescribed steps is doomed to mediocrity and failure." We agree with Pertschuk's sentiment and believe that it is a good reminder for the application of virtually all health promotion interventions. At the same time, however, this call for creativity should not be taken as a diminution of the importance of careful analysis, the application of theory, and sound management. On the contrary, creativity in public health is expressed by combining thoughtful judgment with the freedom to use one's imagination; it is not expressed by the routinized application of a prescribed, one-size-fits-all "cookbook" program.

As implied by these seven ideas, by the time practitioners reach the point at which they are making decisions about intervention tactics, their understanding of the priority health issues and their likely causes should be well established.

The remainder of this chapter is divided into two sections. The first section highlights some of the key aspects of three categories of tactics that have been demonstrated to be effective as parts of a population-based health promotion approach: health communications, media advocacy, and policy tactics. The discussion of policy tactics is presented within the context of a specific problem: tobacco consumption.

The second section describes an emerging methodology that combines computer technology and behavioral theory: tailoring. Globally, health promotion programs have become an increasingly important part of health care planning, policymaking, and delivery. Properly implemented, tailoring methodology offers practitioners the opportunity to combine the specificity of individualized assessments with the efficiency of computer technology to reach large numbers of people with health information that is relevant to them.

HEALTH COMMUNICATIONS, MEDIA ADVOCACY, AND POLICY TACTICS

Health Communications: Follow the Signposts

What do you call it when you exchange thoughts and information with someone? Communication, of course! The Latin root for the word communication is *communicare,* meaning "to make common." As used in the context of public health and health promotion, the concept of health communication certainly incorporates the intuitive objective of making sound health information "common" among all people. However, it also incorporates another important element: analysis. By analysis, we mean the systematic examination and interpretation of information in order to make informed decisions—specifically, decisions about what messages to share, with whom to share them, the most efficient ways to share them, and the most appropriate channels through which they can be disseminated. Without such systematic analysis, health communication efforts run the risk of being driven by opinions (which may not be true), anecdotes (which may not be typical), or stories (which may not be accurate).

Effective practitioners don't guess at the actions they should take; they make decisions. Their decisions are informed by their knowledge of what has gone on in the past and what is going on around them in the present. Effective practitioners are empowered to the extent that they have and use relevant information.

We think that one of the simple keys to taking a systematic approach to health communication is knowing which questions to ask. Based on selective doses of our own experiences and borrowing liberally from some of our favorite resources,[4] we offer the following sequence of health communication "signposts," framed as questions. In seeking responses to these commonsense questions, practitioners will generate most of the information they will need to make informed and insightful decisions.[5]

Signpost 1: What Can Health Communications Do for You?

As you consider the use of health communications, keep in mind that this approach, like all health promotion tactics, has its strengths and weaknesses.

Here are some things that health communication tactics *can* accomplish:

- increase public awareness of a health issue, problem, or solution
- stimulate individuals' reexamination of positive shifts in health-related attitudes
- demonstrate or illustrate skills
- bring to light key health issues to increase public demand for action on those issues
- reinforce knowledge, attitudes, or behavior

Here are some things that health communication tactics are *not* likely to accomplish:

- produce behavior change without supportive program components
- be equally effective in addressing all issues or relaying all messages
- compensate for a lack of essential staff

Suppose that you are involved in a breast cancer early-detection program and one of the key objectives of the program is to increase by 50 percent the number of women age 50 and older in your service area who have had a screening mammogram. The decision as to whether a given health communication tactic should be a part of your overall intervention strategy will obviously be informed by data you have gathered in prior planning steps. This information could include the prevalence of screening mammograms among women over 50 by level of education, income, and locale; the attitudes of physicians regarding the importance of screening mammograms in their practices; and the perceptions of women about the risks, benefits, costs, availability and accessibility of screening services. In combination, the next two signposts can help you decide which pieces of information are most relevant.

Signpost 2: With Whom Are You Trying to Communicate?

In the breast cancer screening example, the target group might be all women over 50, or the subset of women over 50 who have not had a mammogram. However, it might be husbands, friends, or family members of women over 50 who have not had a mammogram. It could also be primary-care physicians, owners of businesses in the service area that serve women over 50, or some combination of all of these.

In the language of market research, determining specifically who your audience is to be is called *segmenting the market*. Once you have determined the audience (segment) to be reached, your probe for information continues with an *audience analysis*. In this process, you are trying to become aware of the characteristics you need to take into account if you are to make effective contact with the group in question.

Why is such analysis necessary? Because social marketing theory and empirical evidence confirm what common sense tells us: not everyone responds the same way to the same message.[6] Depending upon the diversity and size of the group, important characteristics might include age, sex, level of education, current level of awareness about (and attitudes toward) the problem, occupation, geographic location, and cultural orientation. Whether the group in question consists of Pakistani villagers at risk of infection from dracunculiasis (guinea worm disease) or influential business leaders with the power to change environmental policies, the need for specific information, and the process to obtain it, remains the same.

Some communications experts suggest that there is merit in dividing audiences into subgroups. For example, Figure 6.2 displays five audiences relevant to a priority health problem in all developing countries: diarrheal disease. Note that two groups (mothers and caretakers of children age zero to four; and community elders, leaders, shopkeepers, and teachers) have been designated as the *primary* audience and the remaining three groups as the *secondary* audiences. The positioning of the secondary audiences purposefully reflects their respective relationships with the primary audience. As such, it provides us with two graphic reminders:

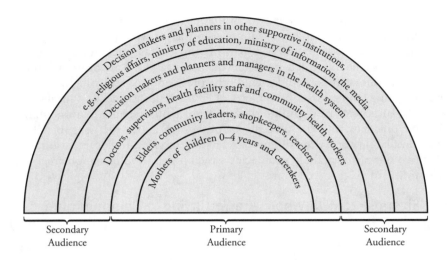

Secondary Audience   Primary Audience   Secondary Audience

FIGURE 6.2 Primary and Secondary Audiences for Oral Rehydration

1. We need to pay heed to secondary audiences because they can and often do function as channels of communication to other secondary audiences and to the primary audience. (See signpost 4 for additional details on channels of communication.)

2. In addition to the primary audience, secondary audiences may also be a priority for communications attention. Consider the frontline staff and medical practitioners in the third-tier semicircle in Figure 6.2. Although they may be quite skilled in providing medical services, they may not perceive the merits of taking the time (or they may lack the ability) to communicate the needs and benefits of oral rehydration therapy (ORT), proper feeding, and preventive practices to those they are serving.

Signpost 3: What Does It Cost Your Audience to Hear Your Message?

In consumer marketing, the price of a particular product is usually clear to both the customer and the marketer because it has a specific dollar value assigned to it—one that the consumer can either accept or reject. Of course, many factors affect whether a consumer will buy a particular product (hence the advertising industry!). Nevertheless, consumer transactions generally involve exchanging your hard-earned cash for something that you really want or need, or that someone has convinced you that you really want or need. The price (along with the inconvenience of getting to the store, etc.) represents the cost to you. Thus, the act of purchasing a product is a way of saying that you think it's worthwhile.

    In health communications, the costs are much murkier, and so are the benefits or incentives. Instead of asking your audience to fork over cash for something they want or need—something that will give them immediate pleasure and satisfaction—you are often asking them to do the opposite. You may be asking them to try something uncomfortable, inconvenient, unfamiliar, and/or frightening, for which there may not be immediate benefits. In fact, the immediate effects may be quite discouraging! Quitting smoking, getting a mammogram, and changing one's diet or exercise patterns all come to mind as examples of health behaviors that have a high sticker price for a given audience.

In analyzing your audience segments and designing your messages, make sure that you understand the "costs" that your audiences perceive. That understanding becomes the grounds upon which you can frame messages to clarify misconceptions, allay fears, or both.

Signpost 4: What Do You Want to Say?

The task of determining with whom you want to communicate is virtually inseparable from the task of determining the most appropriate message to communicate. The goal here is to have a clear understanding of what it is you want the audience in question to do as a result of its exposure to the message. For example, in terms of your ultimate project goal, are you trying to achieve shifts among the audience in: visits to health care providers; calls to a hotline number; reading specific literature; using a certain product; setting aside time to exercise?

Specificity is important in selecting a message. For example, urging a population of women in Los Angeles to "Get a mammogram," or a group of villagers in Ghana to "Drink clean water," may be too general. More specific messages, such as, "Ask a health care provider whether you should have a mammogram," or, "Drink water that has been passed through a proper filter," may be more realistic and appropriate.

Again, your initial ideas about the intent and content of the message will be informed by information gleaned during earlier planning. Once you have framed your initial idea for messages, social marketing research experts would encourage you to pretest those ideas to ensure that the audience for whom they are intended will see them as interesting, memorable, understandable, acceptable, relevant to their situation, and credible.

An excellent academic resource describing both the theory and methods of designing health messages is a book by that title: *Designing Health Messages,* edited by Maibach and Parrott.[8] It contains detailed accounts and many examples of message design and testing efforts. Included in this publication is a description by Lefebvre and his colleagues[9] of the research that went into the formulation of some of the messages in the "5 a Day for Better Health" program campaign carried out by the National Cancer Institute.[10] After acknowledging that the costs for original market research and analysis can be potentially prohibitive for large-scale campaigns, they explain how, by searching and analyzing data from secondary sources, they were able to obtain the information required to design effective messages at a much lower cost. In this instance, secondary sources included marketing databases that had been established and were periodically updated by various companies, associations, and organizations. We highlight this point to alert practitioners to the possibility that as the technology for creating and tracking consumer databases becomes more refined, such databases (at reasonable costs) are likely to become more available and accessible for health communication planning.

That said, most health promotion workers, especially those who serve in small or remote areas, will have to conduct their own customized message and materials testing, instead of relying on secondary sources. A variety of methods (singly or in combination) can be used to pretest messages and materials. These include questionnaires, focus groups, theater testing, central-location intercept interviews, and readability testing. The U.S. National Institutes of Health publication, *Making Health Communications Work: A Planner's Guide,* is a good source of background information on health communications, and contains very clear and practical descriptions of these basic pretesting methods.

Signpost 5: How Will the Message Get to Your Audience?

Market researchers define the term *channel* simply as the vehicle that transmits a message from a source to a receiver.[11] Here are some examples of channels that community health promotion practitioners might consider:

- interpersonal or face-to-face interaction (teacher to student, parent to child, physician to patient)
- planned group meetings or gatherings (workplaces, communities of faith, classrooms)
- the community (libraries, periodic civic events, local government organizations, shopping centers and malls)
- mass media (radio, television, newspapers, magazines, newsletters, direct mail, billboards)
- the Internet (electronic mail, Web pages, bulletin boards)
- organizations or associations (volunteer health organizations, service organizations, professional societies)

Here are three basic questions to ask prior to making your choices about the channels most appropriate for your situation:

- Given the budgetary, personnel, and time resources available to you, is the channel feasible?
- Will the audience perceive this channel to be credible?

- Does the proposed channel fit the purpose of the health communication; that is, if your goal is to trigger a new behavior, is there any evidence that use of this channel will work?

Recall that we earlier defined *channel* as a vehicle through which a source sends a message to a receiver. Of course, sometimes the source (also referred to as the sender) and the channel are one and the same, for example, a parent communicating with a child, or vice versa, as in the case of school health programs that feature children communicating health ideas to their parents. We highlight this overlap to alert practitioners to the reality that a health communication effort is likely to be severely compromised if the receiver has doubts about or conflicts with the sender or source.

We found this to be true based on our effort to evaluate the American Cancer Society's Reach to Recovery Program.[12] Reach to Recovery is a service program wherein volunteers provide postsurgical support to women who have undergone surgery for breast cancer. The goal of the program is to assist patients to a healthful adjustment to their surgery and to help them get on with normal lives. The volunteers in this program are women who themselves have experienced and made healthful adjustments to breast cancer surgery. The importance of the credibility of the volunteers in this program was best reflected in this quote from a patient in Pennsylvania:

> When a *Reach* volunteer walks into that hospital room, looking happy and balanced, she sends a message of hope to that patient—the kind of hope that neither the physician nor nurse can provide.

However, an important observation in this evaluation was that the credibility of having had the same experience (*e.g.,* breast cancer surgery) was insufficient when there were cultural or ethnic differences between the volunteer and the patient. In addition, on-site interviews revealed that in some instances, even the standard visit approach seemed to be incompatible. For example, it was reported that in one-on-one visits, Hispanic women in Los Angeles felt uncomfortable because they were asked to disclose intimate information to a "stranger." Further inquiry revealed that a "support group" approach in places that the patient perceived to be friendly surroundings was much more acceptable.

Such accounts serve to remind us not to lose sight of the commonsense courtesy inherent when you are consciously respectful of cultural differences. They also remind us why the community is the center of gravity for health promotion. Decisions about priorities and strategies for social change are best made as close as possible to where people work, live, and go to school.[13] Communities are relevant, and it is precisely because community health promotion practitioners work amid such relevance that they have so much potential for making a difference.

That said, the Australian health promotion expert Simon Chapman offers us this cautionary note about the inherent superiority of one approach over another:

> The top down or "done to" approach is frequently depicted as heinous and Stalinist, whereas "done with" approaches are seen as politically correct and mandatory. This dichotomy is far too simplistic: there are many examples where top down/done to/upstream strategies in health promotion (so-called passive prevention strategies), initiated by non-consulting health professionals, have been greeted warmly by the public and shown to have benefited public health in important ways. Random breath testing, comprehensive food labeling, Papanicolaou smears, mandatory bicycle crash helmets and vehicle seat belts, fluoridated water supply, taxes on cigarettes and alcohol, vehicle safety checks and standards . . . this list could go on. All these are hardly popular in the sense that they cause people to take to the streets, many involve things being "done to" people, many have been introduced with next to no involvement or loud expressions of interest by consumers, yet many of them are the success stories of modern public health.[14]

Media Advocacy:
Addressing the "Manufacturers of Illness"

The scientific assessment of the causes of health problems has led us to the understanding that a large portion of disease, death, and disability is associated with identifiable behavioral and environmental factors, many of which are amenable to change. Table 6.1 provides a clear illustration of this point; note that smoking and dietary behaviors account for 33 percent of the total number of deaths per year in the United States.

Analyses that led to the information presented in Table 6.1 suggest that there is substantial public health merit in seeking to alert the public to the preventable nature of the leading causes of death. In the language of supply and demand, the main focus of this approach has been on the demand side: (1) strengthening the capacity (knowledge, healthful practices) of those at risk, and (2) creating surroundings conducive to health. The health communications tactics described in the previous section are designed to address these important demand factors.

At the same time, it is clear that some of the important causes of today's priority health problems may fall outside the lens of our traditional epidemiologic focus. For example, although their role in ill health is well recognized by public health officials, corporations that produce tobacco, alcohol, handguns, and automatic weapons are not classified in terms of relative

TABLE 6.1   Actual Leading Causes of Death in the United States

Cause	Number	% of Total
Tobacco	400,000	19
Diet/activity patterns	300,000	14
Alcohol	100,000	5
Microbial agents	90,000	4
Toxic agents	60,000	3
Sexual behaviors	40,000	2
Firearms	35,000	2
Illicit drug use	25,000	1
Motor vehicles	20,000	<1

Source: McGinnis MJ, Foege WH. Actual causes of death in the United States. *Journal of the American Medical Association.* 1993;270:2207–2212.

risk. These "manufacturers of illness" represent the supply side of the equation because they produce and aggressively market products with little or no regard for their negative effects on health.[15]

Common sense should tell us that a health promotion program aimed at the demand side while ignoring the supply side is bound to be weaker than a program that systematically addresses both. Doesn't it seem futile to teach youth about tobacco-, alcohol-, and drug-abuse prevention in a community where cigarettes, alcohol, and drugs can be purchased as easily as groceries? Does it make sense to withhold our efforts to inform and educate the public about healthful eating while we simultaneously undertake the long-range process of developing policies that will make low-fat dairy products available and accessible?

Enter Media Advocacy and Politics

We emphasize media advocacy precisely because its aim is to address the evasive, often political supply aspect of health problems. Practitioners should keep in mind the important distinction between health communications (social marketing) and media advocacy. While both employ the media, the former seeks to promote personal responsibility and lifestyle change, and the latter seeks to attain the implementation of healthful policy.

The word *advocacy* means to defend, support, or champion a person or cause. It is a word that connotes passion and action. Although advocates are respectful of convention, it is not at all unusual for them to choose to support their cause over adherence to a convention. This approach differs in character from the standard practice of planning health promotion and disease prevention programs, which is grounded in epidemiology, the basic science of public health. Epidemiologic analysis gives us clues about the causal chain of events that lead to a particular health problem; in turn, this knowledge serves to guide us in the formulation of prevention and health promotion programs.

The Chapter 4 case story, "The Court of Public Opinion," made the point that public health work is political. Decisions are political whenever limited public resources are to be distributed and those involved in the decision-making process are not in agreement about who should get what. For example, suppose you are a member of a community council, and the council members are responsible for annual budget decisions for all community services. Suppose further that you are convinced that the schools need a financial boost, but you are uncertain about the needs of four other departments: roads, police, parks and recreation, and public health. You are a sincere, hardworking, busy person and you find little time for studying the many issues in front of you. Your support is sought by all of these groups. A trusted good friend of the family has encouraged you to take a special look at the business benefits that would occur if the parks and recreation department's lake revitalization project were funded. Can't you almost feel the political pull in that situation?

The reality is that politics are ubiquitous. The challenge for the public health community in general, and health promotion workers in particular, is to acknowledge that reality and to work efficiently and ethically within it. The famous British public health scholar Geoffrey Rose was most sensitive to this issue and offered this wisdom:

> Their [politicians'] agenda is complex and mostly hidden from public scrutiny. This is unfortunate, because often the public would give higher priority to health than those who formulate political policies. Anything which stimulates more public information and debate on health issues is good, not just because it may lead to healthier choices by individuals, but also because it earns a higher place for health issues on the political agenda. In the long run, this is probably the most important achievement of health education.[16]

Some Practical First Steps

Current health promotion literature offers rich and creative guidance on the implementation of media advocacy; we strongly urge practitioners to consult these existing resources for added depth and detail on the process.[17] In this section we highlight a few practical issues that we hope will help practitioners get their teeth into media advocacy.

Larry Wallack and Lori Dorfman are public health professionals whose lucid writing and training efforts have done much to enhance our awareness and understanding of media advocacy.[18] To help give audiences a grasp of what media advocacy is about, they often use this quote attributed to Scoop Nisker, of KFOG radio in San Francisco: "If you don't like the news, go out and make some of your own!"

In effect, Nisker is saying several things here: (1) don't whine—it won't get you anywhere; (2) identify the "news" you want the public to attend to; and (3) take the initiative and action necessary to get the news to the public. Media advocacy refers to the use of mass media as a means of heightening the public's awareness of a problem and providing them with a means to take legitimate action to address that problem.

We have often thought that having media advocacy skills is like having access to a powerful searchlight that illuminates key unattended public health issues. Since the issues in question are often those that special interests may want to obscure or misrepresent, one important political result of bringing those issues into full public light is that decision makers are likely to feel uncomfortable if they ignore them.

As in undertaking any organized plan, it is important to be clear on what you want to accomplish.[19] Following are three preliminary steps to help practitioners initiate a media advocacy effort.

Step 1: Determine what your group's policy goal is—what do you want to happen?   Let us suppose that the issue in question is youth violence. Your options might include:

- limit handgun availability
- limit alcohol availability
- increase employment opportunities for youth

Key point: Research your options carefully and be prepared to justify your policy actions for health improvement on the basis of empirical evidence.

Step 2: Determine who your target(s) will be—to whom do you want to speak? When this person, group, or organization speaks, will people listen?   In most health promotion interventions, the target audience consists of those persons at risk of a problem: teen smokers, women over age 50 who have not had a mammogram, children age five to ten who walk in a heavy traffic area. In media advocacy, there are three potential target audiences in descending order of importance: (1) a primary target consisting of the person or group with the power to make a policy change; (2) a secondary target consisting of those who can be mobilized to influence those with the power to make the change; and (3) the general population.

Primary targets might include:

- the city council
- the mayor
- business leaders

Secondary targets might include:

- advocacy groups
- professional societies
- well-known, respected community leaders

Key point: Be specific and focused on your target audience.

Step 3: Be sure your message or story is clear. All too frequently we hear that the media "just didn't get the story right!" While it is quite possible that they didn't, it is probably more likely that at least part of the problem can be attributed to a failure on the part of the advocate to make the message or story clear. To help us sharpen the clarity of our message, Wallack and Dorfman ask us to pay particular attention to three elements of our communication with the media:

1. **Be clear about the statement of concern:** "Tobacco is everywhere, and youth are especially at risk because . . ."
2. **Highlight a value dimension:** Tobacco companies are making economic profit with literally no regard to the unnecessary death, disease, and disability they cause.
3. **State the policy objective:** Stores that sell tobacco to minors will be fined $5,000 per incident.

Key point: Getting the media's attention is an important point, but don't stop there; have a specific message ready once you've gotten their attention! Be prepared to help them write their script if asked.

Finally, throughout the process of planning a media advocacy effort, responsible practitioners will create a system of monitoring the progress and effects of all of these steps. Routine analysis and discussion of such information among members of your planning team is the most efficient means of assessing how you are progressing and, more important, what changes are necessary to keep you on course.

If You Don't "Frame It" Correctly,
They Aren't Likely to Get It!

The effective application of media advocacy is dependent upon a good understanding of the concept of *framing.* In this age of information, we can all identify with the struggle of having to sift through the never-ending attempts to get our attention—e-mail, faxes, meetings, telephone solicitations, surveys, mail-order catalogs, newspaper headlines; the list seems endless. Obviously, what we attend to will depend on our perceived needs and interests—that is, we are likely to pay attention to information that is packaged, or framed, in a context that interests us. Wallack and Dorfman suggest that media advocacy is organized around two complementary frames: framing for *access* and framing for *content.* In both cases the broad concept remains the same: package your information so that those for whom it is intended will pay attention.

Framing for Access. *Framing for access* means preparing your story in such a way that you maximize your chances of getting access to the media. If you took the time to make a listing of the stories covered on the local and network television and radio news programs, you would note that virtually all of the programs cover the same stories. Obtaining this kind of broad and repeated exposure for a critical health issue is a first-level objective of media advocacy.

As practitioners make plans to gain access to the media, the most fundamental idea we can offer is this: Think like a reporter. Make an appointment with a TV, radio, or newspaper reporter and simply ask some straightforward questions:

How do you gather news?

How do you determine what stories will be aired or printed?

What can I give you that will make your job easier?

Framing for Content. *Framing for content* means preparing a story in such a way that it prompts the target audience to acknowledge that any serious consideration of a solution to the problem must go beyond the individuals or victims involved, to include policy actions that can influence the environmental/social conditions that made the problem possible in the first place.

The Key: Anticipation

Great athletes are also great anticipators. For example, effective shortstops in baseball anticipate that every ball will be hit to them; with full knowledge of how many people are on base, how many outs there are, what kind of pitch the pitcher is going to deliver, the speed of the runners, and the teams' defensive strengths and weaknesses, the shortstop calculates all of the possible contingencies *before* they occur. Because they are disciplined to anticipate so well, great athletes never seem to hesitate or give the appearance that they are in doubt. When asked why he always seemed to be in the right place at the right time, hockey star Wayne Gretzky replied simply, "I skate to where I think the puck will be!"

Practitioners whose mental model of health promotion includes media advocacy also anticipate well. They look for and scan stories and events for their advocacy potential—in fact, for the busy practitioner in the field, piggybacking, or tying your issue to a breaking news story, may constitute the best opportunity to attract news coverage. Editorial commentaries, letters to the editor, op-ed pieces, and talk show appearances can provide an effective and timely means for obtaining coverage.[20]

Let's consider how you might apply the idea of piggybacking in combination with the notion of framing for content described earlier. Say that you and your health promotion colleagues in the community of San Pablo having been working to enhance your community's appreciation for the reality that the tobacco problem cannot be seriously addressed without taking action on the root source of the problem: the tobacco industry. One morning you pick up a copy of the *San Pablo Daily News* to discover that the CDC has released findings from its Youth Risk Behavior Survey indicating that smoking prevalence among youth, especially girls, has increased significantly over the past two years. Two days later, the news media is saturated with the tragic story of an airline crash in Florida, killing 110 people. Serious questions are raised about the responsibility of the airline with regard to its concern for and implementation of safety practices.

You and your colleagues see the opportunity to reframe these two stories to call the community's attention to your message. You create this op-ed piece for submission to the *San Pablo Daily News*:

We wonder . . .

Let's give credit where credit is due. The tobacco industry is *really* good—their sharply focused marketing and sales strategies set the standard for the business world. They know *precisely* what their product can do, and they know who is using it now and who will be using it in the future. Their stockholders enjoy a huge profit on their investment. The tobacco industry is really good. That their product is both addictive and lethal matters not, because the power of profit is the highest canon by which questions of ethics are decided in a world run by business.

RJR Nabisco, Phillip Morris, Brown and Williamson, and Liggett are absolutely convinced that with the support of freedom-loving Americans like you and me, they will continue to justify their right to make billions of dollars of profit regardless of the cost to others.

Such is the chilling, calculated arrogance of the tobacco industry.

Every day, tobacco companies make a conscious decision to make money by the aggressive global marketing of an addictive, lethal product. In spite of the warnings from the world's scientific community (over 50,000 studies document the causal effects of tobacco consumption on death, disease, and disability), the captains of the tobacco industry brazenly hawk products that continue to kill millions of human beings each year—and this is done in the name of freedom and the right to earn money. Through their potent lobby, tobacco companies have used their corporate muscle to influence U.S. trade representatives to force open foreign markets—and in the process, they shamelessly attack and ridicule the anti-tobacco health protection measures of those nations as "unfair trade barriers."

To put the lethal impact of tobacco into perspective, consider the tragic ValuJet crash in Florida, which resulted in the loss of 110 lives. The airline's corporate leaders and personnel are shocked and saddened, and have vowed to make the investments necessary to correct what went awry. Conversely, tobacco causes the equivalent of ten ValuJet crashes *every day* in the United States. And how does the tobacco industry respond to such news? First, they deny any wrongdoing and tell us, under oath and with a straight face, that they have no knowledge that their product is either addictive or lethal. Then, in the name of freedom, they point to the public, saying in effect, "Look, this is a free country and people have a right to choose."

Through clever advertising and marketing, much of which is aimed at youth, they make the choice an easy one. Last month we saw the latest data: A new CDC study shows that 35 percent of American youth are now smokers—that's up from 28 percent in 1991. The tobacco industry is celebrating this as a victory and a harbinger of things to come! How can the "right" to promote and earn profit from a product that kills have meaning in a free and civil society? Conspicuously missing from the tobacco industry's rhetoric on rights is the moral principle of social responsibility. But then, according to the Nobel Prize–winning economist Milton Friedman social responsibility has no place in good business:

> Few trends could so thoroughly undermine the very foundations of our free society as the acceptance by corporate officials of a social responsibility other than to make as much money for their shareholders as possible.
>
> —Friedman M, Friedman RD.
> *Capitalism and Freedom.*
> Chicago: University of Chicago Press; 1962.

This rhetoric artfully links the drive to make as much money as possible to the powerful moral value of freedom, while claiming that the connection between economic gain and freedom would be compromised if corporate leaders were socially responsible. The picture is unambiguous: tobacco corporations care about profits, not human beings. The tobacco issue is not about individual rights, free choice, tolerance of minority views, or crop diversification. It is about the human vice—greed— deliberately stoking the fires of a human failing—addiction.

We wonder . . . are any citizens of San Pablo personally offended by this arrogance? How many tobacco company stockholders really understand what they are investing in? At what point do we all begin acting like citizens and say enough is enough? Why can't we start right here in San Pablo? We wonder. . . .

Some Final Questions

Practitioners whose mental model of health promotion includes a command of advocacy skills are more likely to anticipate and seize opportunities and then effectively translate them into media advocacy applications. Interviews with practitioners who have effectively applied media advocacy have inspired us to create the following scenario, followed by a series of circumstances and questions designed to stimulate your thinking about the options afforded you to get your message framed and "out there."

Scenario: For some time, you have been working for policy action that addresses the fact that youth in Newbury have easy access to alcohol. Existing laws are not enforced.

News Story: The citizens of Newbury today are mourning the death and serious injury of six teenagers from their community. Last night, six teenagers in a six-passenger sports vehicle were returning from an early-evening party at Old Mountain. They had been celebrating their upcoming graduation from high school. There was dancing, singing, and volleyball at the party—and there was also plenty of cold beer. All of the passengers in the car had been drinking, including the driver. Eyewitnesses in the car behind the victims indicated that it appeared as if the driver lost control of his car on a sharp turn and hit a tree near the roadside. Two of the teenagers were killed and four were injured, three seriously. [Initially, the media frames this story around the notion that teens and parents need to take more responsibility to prevent alcohol-related problems.]

Situation 1: Knowing that you work on this issue, a reporter from the Newbury paper contacts you and asks for your comment.

- What do you say?
- Do you have a prepared statement?
- Do you have a list of reputable, credible local resource people who are willing to help make and support your point of view?

- Do you have to clear your comments to the media through your supervisor, the agency public relations office, or your agency director?
- Are you prepared to point to successful policy actions other communities have taken to address this issue?

Situation 2:   The media contacts you specifically to comment on (you suspect they would like you to support) their contention that this is yet another example of the deterioration of family responsibility.

- What do you say?
- Did you anticipate this kind of confirmation request, and are you prepared to frame your response to get your message across?
- Again, are you prepared to refer them to reputable citizens who are willing to help make and support your point of view?

Situation 3:   The media contacts your agency director for a comment.

- Did you anticipate your director being called?
- If so, did you brief your director in advance and leave him or her some written backup material?
- Does your director understand that he or she is not alone in the position you are advocating?

Situation 4:   The media doesn't call you, your director, or any of your colleagues.

This means that the initiative for making contact with the media about this story shifts to you.

- Prior to this story breaking, did you take the time to establish prior relationships with members of the media?
- Have you obtained the appropriate clearance to make contact with the media?
- Have you prepared a written account that "frames" the story around the issues of youth access to alcohol?

Applying Policy and Regulatory Approaches: A Tobacco Example

The integration of policy actions into a health promotion will strengthen that program in two ways: first, by the declaration that the issue in question is so important that it merits formal policy support. The second benefit is that of longevity—that is, policy is as difficult to change as it is to implement. Therefore, once the program is in place, the chances of sustaining your health promotion initiative over time are increased.

Because they can have a direct effect upon demand for and access to tobacco, legislative/policy tactics are among the most powerful tools health promotion practitioners can use in their efforts to control tobacco use. In addition, there is evidence that even as an independent action, legislative/policy tactics can significantly reduce tobacco consumption.[21]

However, the use of policy-oriented tactics is a complex and demanding undertaking. It requires careful orchestration and management of a well-organized, well-informed coalition whose membership is both politically savvy and patient. Practitioners must also be prepared for the very real possibility of potential backlash from those who feel that legislative actions infringe upon freedom. In this section, we illustrate how five specific policy-oriented tactics can be orchestrated in combination to help practitioners attain a goal of reducing youth access to tobacco.

To begin with, you will find it useful to ask a series of questions to establish the climate for legislative action within your community. Such questions might include:

1. Have you identified individuals/organizations that could be advocates for tobacco-use control among youth?
2. Have you identified existing legislation regarding tobacco access to minors and retail tobacco license laws? Is this legislation enforced?
3. Have you identified a legislative outcome that you would like to see occur?
4. Are youth particularly targeted within your community? Are any tobacco billboards located within 1,000 feet of your schools?

Tactic A: Establishing the Basic Groundwork

Recommended actions to take:

1. Conduct tobacco purchase surveys to determine the extent and magnitude of the problem within your community.
2. Obtain information on how and where minors get tobacco in your community or surrounding areas.
3. Prepare information that clearly describes the nature of the problem; use informal group testing to determine the extent to which citizens find the information you have prepared to be understandable and worth their attention.

Tactic B: Modify the Selling Practices of Merchants

Recommended actions to take:

1. As a first step, use existing communication channels to inform merchants, civic groups, and all relevant community organizations about the problem, with emphasis on where and how youth get tobacco.

2. Encourage the local media to cover the problem of easy access to an addictive agent.

3. Conduct a merchant education program. Use a balanced approach, emphasizing civic responsibility and community benefits as well as the potential for penalties to owners, license suspension, and legal precedents for civil lawsuits against those in violation of sales-to-minors laws.

4. Create and post clever warning signs at all points of purchase.

5. Identify merchants whose practice it is *not* to sell tobacco to minors and make this information widely known as a healthful establishment (an honor similar to the *Good Housekeeping* seal of approval).

6. Identify merchants who *do* sell tobacco to minors and make this information widely known.

7. Promote the positive use of ID checks for all tobacco sales.

Tactic C: Increase Enforcement of Existing Laws Prohibiting Sales to Minors

Recommended actions to take:

1. If law enforcement agencies in your community do not consider enforcement of youth access laws to be a priority, explore the possibility of having an alternative agency so designated—the public health department, for example.

2. Create a legitimate mechanism for citizens to file complaints against non-compliant merchants.

3. Create compliance checks and undercover buying operations (UBOs). These use underage inspectors, accompanied by adult chaperons, who attempt to purchase tobacco products. UBOs do not result in any penalty to merchants; rather they serve to demonstrate the extent of the problem, warn merchants, and constitute a very real precursor to enforcement.

4. Organize a community coalition to put pressure (through a public demonstration or the media) on relevant authorities to strengthen their enforcement practices.

5. Persuade law enforcement agencies to consider a "three strikes and you're out" policy for retail stores that consistently violate retail license laws and sales-to-minors laws. If enacted, this would mean that after three confirmed violations, retailers would have their license revoked or face other serious penalties.

6. Promote policies and community standards that prohibit the positioning of tobacco in easy-access places, such as in vending machines or on countertops in retail stores. In communities where this practice is illegal, establish fines and penalties for those establishments that continue to sell tobacco products to minors through vending machines.

7. Establish a standard coalition procedure in which members of your tobacco-use control coalition establish a process to routinely communicate with politicians, in order to remain informed about tobacco legislation, as well as to inform the politicians about your views and goals.

Tactic D: Oppose Tobacco Advertising

Approximately 400,000 people die each year from tobacco-related causes; 1.5 million more Americans quit smoking each year. Thus, the tobacco industry must attract 2 million new smokers each year to maintain its market. Youth are particularly vulnerable to tobacco advertising and promotion. The tobacco industry is known for using attractive models in adventurous landscapes in advertisements, as well as promotional giveaways such as T-shirts, Frisbees, and coupons.

Additionally, the tobacco industry specifically targets ethnic groups and women. Tobacco companies contribute extensively to political, social, and artistic organizations such as the Congressional Black Caucus, the National Women's Political Caucus, the Kool Jazz Festival, and Cinco de Mayo celebrations. A notorious example of marketing specifically to a particular group was the introduction of Uptown cigarettes, targeted to African-American populations. A community coalition successfully fought test-marketing in their area. In another case, women's groups were enraged when the tobacco industry introduced Dakota cigarettes, which targeted young "virile" females. Other evidence: One-third of the billboards in New Orleans are located within one-half mile of the city's low-income federal housing projects. Seventy percent of the billboards in Baltimore advertise alcohol and tobacco; three-fourths of those are in predominantly African-American neighborhoods.

Before taking action, consider areas that are specifically targeted within your community or determine areas of improvement.

- Are tobacco billboards located near schools within your community?
- Are events that target large numbers of youth or other groups with limited access to information about the hazards of tobacco consumption sponsored by tobacco companies?
- Are there disproportionate numbers of tobacco billboards in certain segments of your community?

Recommended actions to take:

1. Orchestrate a campaign calling for the following:
   - a ban on the distribution of free tobacco samples or coupons for free samples through the mail or on property accessible to the general public
   - a ban on tobacco advertising on public transit vehicles and in airports, train stations, and bus shelters.

2. Write a sample policy that prohibits tobacco advertising in public facilities such as fairgrounds and sports facilities.

3. Lobby public officials to create smoke-free zones in public areas (such as airports, restaurants, and train stations).

4. Encourage citizens not to patronize facilities using tobacco advertising. (For example, a tobacco-use control coalition in California pressured county fair organizers to drop Phillip Morris as a sponsor. After the issue was widely covered by the media, the fair's board prohibited Marlboro's promotional activities, and Phillip Morris pulled out as a sponsor.)

5. Call to the attention of local leaders the fact that cigarette advertising that uses cartoon characters, such as "Joe Camel," is intended to reach young audiences and children. Standards should prohibit advertising that appeals to this vulnerable population. (A school or church group of children could write letters to local leaders.)

6. Lobby public officials to promote mandatory counteradvertising legislation.

7. Encourage public officials to eliminate the tax deductibility of tobacco advertising expenses.

8. Pressure legislators to enforce existing advertising laws (if any). Document violations of existing laws and failure to enforce those laws.

9. Strive for the removal of all tobacco advertisements within 1,000 feet of a school.

10. Encourage alternative sponsorship of athletic, artistic, cultural, or musical events.

11. Lobby for legislation that reduces the number of tobacco advertisements on billboards or that ensures as many healthy messages as tobacco advertisements.

How to lobby for change:

1. Communicate with or educate decision makers and the general public about the importance of tobacco-use control policies.

2. Advocate for specific policies considered by nonlegislative groups (school boards, state boards of health).

3. Advocate for issues among audiences such as state attorneys general, regulatory authorities, or police authorities for more effective law enforcement or regulation.

4. Aim advocacy actions at government executives (such as mayors and governors).

5. Find out death rates due to coronary heart disease, lung cancer, and bronchitis in your community. Contact local cancer registries or birth/death registries.

6. Find out the prevalence of smokers in your community.

7. Call your legislators and ask what they are going to do about the preventable deaths that are occurring in their districts. They're losing valuable voters!

Effective lobbying is made up of the following components:

- Legislative liaison with the coalition
- Willing legislators
- Organized strategy
- Focused message
- Supportive coalition
- Legislative briefings
- Local events for legislators
- Press development

Tactic E: Economic Incentives

Recommended actions to take:

1. Build a coalition to support raising the cigarette excise tax.
2. Change insurance policies to reward nonsmokers by:
   a. meeting with local business representatives to urge them to provide nonsmoker discounts for employees, and
   b. meeting with local insurance companies to request that they offer reimbursement for smoking-cessation programs.
3. Encourage boycotts of nontobacco products produced by tobacco companies such as RJR Nabisco (for example, Oreo cookies and other food products).

TAILORING: COMBINING TECHNOLOGY WITH THEORY

What Is Tailoring?

Have you ever bought a pair of shoes that seemed to fit in the store, but led to excruciating pain once you tried to walk around in them for a few hours? What about shoes that always give you a blister on that one toe? And how often do you buy a pair of shoes by mail, without trying them on?

When you stop to think about it, shoes seem like an unlikely product to make in mass quantities, despite the many varieties available to us. After all, our feet are all a little bit different—different sizes, shapes, arches, toes, and widths. The same size in one brand may not be exactly right in another brand. For some of us, our two feet aren't even exactly the same size! In fact, we would all be a lot more comfortable if we could afford custom-made shoes. Unfortunately, this is a luxury most of us will never enjoy. Just for a moment, though, imagine what it would be like. Imagine walking into a shoe store. Instead of browsing for some mix of color, shape, and price (and desperately trying to get a salesperson's attention), you would walk up to a computer with a weird foot-shaped pad attached to it. You would step on the pad and let the computer measure every nuance of your foot—not only its length and width, but also the height of your arch, where the ball of your foot falls, the narrowness of your heel, where your ankle bone falls . . . perhaps even whether or not your feet sweat! Then you might answer a few questions about the color and style you are seeking, approve the price, and— *voilà!*—a perfectly fitted pair of shoes would be yours.

Futuristic fantasy? Maybe. But a similar approach is actually being used today in health promotion: using computerized interaction to "tailor" a health promotion program to the unique characteristics of the person for whom it is intended.

We have chosen to highlight tailoring for two reasons: (1) it is a methodological approach that is gaining considerable interest as a means to deliver health education/health promotion with the context of managed care, and (2) it offers a clear, unambiguous illustration of how social, psychological, behavioral, and educational theory is applied in practice.

Health promotion materials are tailored when they are designed in any combination of strategies to reach one specific person and are (1) based on characteristics unique to that person, (2) related to the outcome of interest, and (3) derived from an individual assessment. This concept of trying to get a better "fit" is grounded in sound theory[22] and supported by a growing literature reporting encouraging effects.[23] But just as the cost of tailored clothes and shoes put them out of reach of most people, the opportunity costs of tailoring health messages have caused many community health promotion practitioners to consider the process as having limited potential for reaching large numbers of people; but computer technology in health promotion has changed that.

Tailoring Works!

Studies have shown that assessment-based, computer-generated materials that are tailored to the unique needs and interests of individual subjects can be effective for a variety of health-related behaviors including smoking cessation,[24] dietary management,[25] obtaining screening mammograms,[26] and childhood immunizations.[27] In these studies, subjects who received tailored behavior change information were significantly more likely to make lifestyle changes than were those who received usual medical care, untailored materials, or no messages.

Although tailoring, targeting, and personalizing are all associated with the notion of specificity, they are not synonymous. For example, earlier in this chapter we indicated that materials and messages could be *targeted* based on principles of market segmentation, which seek to identify key demographic characteristics of subgroups within the general population. Properly planned, this approach can lead to the development of educational materials that are more likely to be attended by the target populations; but those materials would not be considered tailored.

Tailored health promotion materials also should not be confused with *personalized* materials. Personalization involves the use of a person's name to draw attention to an untailored message. A common commercial marketing example in the United States is the use of direct-mail tactics for the promotion of popular magazine sales (*e.g.,* "Mary Beth Johnson, you may have already won $2,500,000!").

Both targeted and personalized communications base their messages on demographic factors such as age, race, sex, and name—all of which are unique to the potential receivers of the information. However, the assumption in tailoring is that demographic factors alone are not likely to provide the information sufficient to address complex health behaviors. For example, if you were developing a dietary-change program, which would be more useful to you—knowing the age, race, and sex of participants, or knowing about their specific dietary attitudes, habits, and eating patterns? A computerized tailoring approach enables you to draw on the strengths of both sources of information. In addition, the application of computer technology also lessens the interview burden for the practitioner and the individual.

Tailored communication is grounded in the following assumptions:

- Individual assessment tends to eliminate superfluous information and bring into focus information that is personally relevant to the recipient.

- People pay more attention to information they perceive to be personally relevant.

- Information that draws one's attention is more likely to stimulate or support action than that which does not.

How Are Tailored Materials Created?

The process of creating tailored health promotion materials involves five general tasks:

1. analyzing the problem and understanding its determinants
2. developing an assessment tool to measure a person's status based on these determinants

3. creating tailored messages that address the determinants of the problem

4. developing a database to store participants' responses

5. developing tailoring algorithms that translate participants' responses from the database into tailored messages

We have summarized the major steps in carrying out these tasks in Table 6.2. To act on these steps, health practitioners will need to call on their basic health promotion competencies in behavioral science theory, questionnaire design, and development of educational messages, and combine them with the skills of those capable of creating linked databases and general computer programming.[28]

Since our main purpose in highlighting the process of tailoring is to illustrate how theory directly affects the practitioner's selection of methods, we will focus our attention primarily on the first three steps in the process. See endnote 29 for a brief description of some of the key points of steps 4 and 5 in Table 6.2.

Step 1: Analyze the Problem

As we have emphasized throughout this book, especially in Chapter 3, effective practitioners make it a priority to understand the determinants of the problem they seek to address. Consider again the metaphor of tailored messages being like custom-made shoes. For a shoemaker, the key measurements will vary depending upon the type of shoe and the customer's measurements. Elegant fabrics, lines, and shapes might be required for dress shoes, while durability and comfort are required for sports shoes. The same is true for tailoring health promotion materials: the key "measurements," or determinants, vary depending on the outcome of interest. For example, a tailored program to help participants quit smoking may require an assessment of their readiness to quit[30] or their self-efficacy for quitting.[31] In contrast, tailored materials promoting breast cancer screening might focus on a woman's perceived risk of breast cancer, her beliefs about mammography, and/or the barriers to getting a mammogram that she perceives.

So how do you determine the key variables for a given health problem? First, get familiar with what we already know. Review the research literature describing the factors associated with the promotion of healthful behaviors; this will generate ideas for the determinants to look out for. Globally, the health promotion research literature is a huge information resource, and it is getting better every year. As you scan the literature, see how prominent theories of health-related behavior change previously cited (*e.g.*, the transtheoretical model, the Health Belief Model, self-efficacy and social learning theories, and relapse prevention theory) are used to explain the change process. To help you put all of this into a manageable framework, we suggest that you use the process of identifying the causes described in Chapter 3.

TABLE 6.2   Steps in Carrying Out the Key Tasks for Tailoring Health Promotional Materials

Analyzing the Problem	Developing an Assessment Tool	Creating Tailored Messages	Developing a Database	Developing Tailoring Algorithms
1. Define the problem and target population 2. Identify factors that influence the problem (i.e., determinants) 3. Determine which of these factors are amenable to change 4. Prioritize among candidate determinants (i.e., select variables to be addressed in tailored communication) 5. Set objectives to be achieved by tailored communication	1. Identify or develop questions to measure key determinants 2. Identify potential response choices for each question 3. Prioritize among candidate response choices 4. Determine best method for data collection 5. Pretest assessment tool among members of the target population	1. List assessment questions and response choices to be addressed by tailored messages 2. Identify intervention strategies that could be used to address each possible response choice for each assessment question 3. Determine which strategies can be delivered effectively via tailored messages 4. Develop message concepts describing how each strategy could be communicated in tailored messages 5. Pretest message concepts 6. Create tailored messages that address key message concepts 7. Pretest tailored messages	1. Assign a variable name to each question in the assessment tool 2. Create a variable key that assigns a numeric value to each response choice for each question in the assessment tool 3. Develop a database to store respondents' answers to the assessment questions	1. Create a single message library that contains all tailored messages 2. Assign a different variable name to each tailored message in the library 3. Using the variable names from the questions and tailored messages, write "if/then" logic statements linking the numeric value of each response choice to its corresponding tailored message from the tailoring library 4. Incorporate algorithms into a single computer program that will merge participant responses from the database with messages from the tailoring library 5. Test tailoring program extensively

This process will yield a list of candidate factors to be considered as key determinants of the outcome of interest. To narrow the list, consider which are most changeable, most important (*i.e.,* have the greatest influence on the outcome of interest), and most pertinent for the particular population being addressed. Tailored interventions will be most efficient when this process identifies the fewest number of determinants that predict the greatest amount of change in the outcome of interest. As an example, analyzing the problem of cigarette smoking might reveal the following factors to be important for the outcome of cessation: readiness to quit, level of addiction to nicotine, perceived barriers to quitting, self-efficacy for quitting, motives for quitting, and past experience trying to quit.

Step 2: Develop an Assessment Tool

Because tailored materials are assessment based, a questionnaire or survey must be developed to measure a person's status on each of the factors identified in Step 1. These surveys may be self-administered, administered by an interviewer, or even administered by an interactive computer program. Whatever the format, their distinguishing characteristic is the limited choice of answers to their questions. In order to create all possible tailored messages before the assessment takes place, the response choices to each question must be known. A major part of developing the assessment tool, then, is determining the response choices that will accompany each assessment question.

For efficiency, it will be most helpful if you use the smallest number of response options that are likely to capture the largest percentage of respondents. For example, if 100 smokers were surveyed, they might give fifteen different reasons for wanting to quit smoking. But if 90 of the smokers give one of five reasons, and the remaining 10 each give an entirely different reason, it is probably most practical for your question about motivation to quit to include just those five most common answers. How do you identify the appropriate or most common response choices? Research papers on the topic of interest present such data, as do review articles that summarize existing knowledge about changing a given behavior. In many cases, especially with theoretical variables, questions with established psychometric properties already exist and can be used as is, or modified to meet the needs of the tailoring assessment.

Building on the example from Step 1, responses to an assessment tool for smoking would yield valuable and specific information on such factors as readiness to quit, level of addiction to nicotine, perceived barriers to quitting, self-efficacy for quitting, motives for quitting, and past experience trying to quit and social support. Figure 6.3 provides an example of how responses to these seven factors create an individual profile—you can see that this level of information would be crucial to tailoring smoking-cessation programs and in communicating their robustness to others.

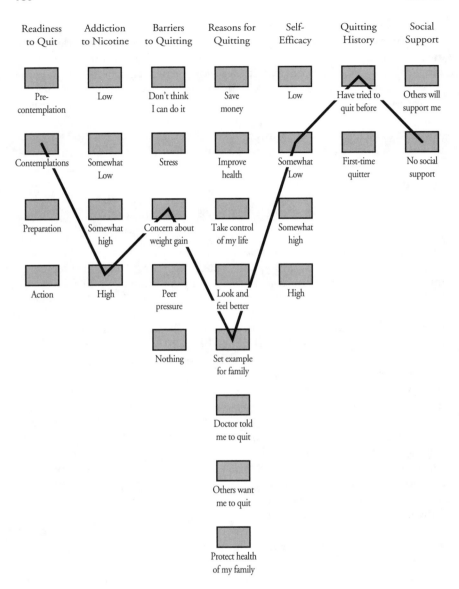

FIGURE 6.3 Individual Profile Generated from a Theory-Based Survey

Step 3: Create Tailored Messages

When you have identified the key determinants of the outcome of interest, the questions to assess those determinants, and the most common response choices for each question, you will have the necessary information to begin

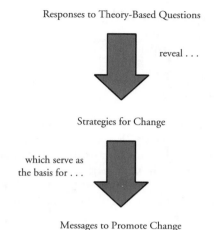

Responses to Theory-Based Questions

reveal . . .

Strategies for Change

which serve as
the basis for . . .

Messages to Promote Change

FIGURE 6.4 How Theory Guides the Tailoring Process

crafting your tailored messages. Recall the references to mental models in earlier chapters. The mental model that guides the process of creating tailored messages provides us with an unambiguous illustration of how theory is used to inform the development of an intervention strategy and, therefore, the tactics needed to carry out that strategy.

Figure 6.4 offers a simple illustration of that process; let's walk through an example to see how it works. Suppose the goal is to provide tailored messages designed to increase physical activity among a population of senior citizens, as might be the case in either a senior citizens' center or a medical practice specializing in geriatrics.

The individuals in question are asked to complete a questionnaire. Each question is grounded in some aspect of theory deemed to be relevant to the goal. For example, consider the following questions:

Yes	No	Not Sure	
☐	☐	☐	Are you interested in improving your level of physical fitness?
Yes	No	Not Sure	
☐	☐	☐	Are you interested in improving your flexibility?

A "Yes" response to these questions would suggest that the respondent is at the contemplation or ready-for-action stage, based on Stages of Change Theory. Not only does this give the planner important information about the individual's readiness for change, it also provides insight into the strategies most likely to be attended to and tried by the respondent. A "Yes" response would also prompt the respondent to answer other questions designed to reveal added information to help in the decision process. For example:

Which of the following would be a barrier to you initiating a physical activity program?

a. I tried before and failed
b. I don't have the time
c. It's too difficult

This question, of course, is derived from the Health Belief Model and addresses the issue of perceived barriers. Each response option acts as a prompt that will point in the direction of theoretically sound and compatible strategies. For example, if the "I tried before and failed" option was selected, there is sound theory, supported by research evidence, to suggest that a strategy promoting skills associated with self-efficacy has a high probability of being effective. Based on this rationale, messages that provide clear guidance on how to establish realistic, attainable goals, how to monitor personal progress, and tips for creating positive self-feedback would all be appropriate.

If the "it's too difficult" option was chosen, it might prompt the following message concept based on physical activity research: *The maximum benefit in cardiorespiratory fitness will be obtained by moving from little or no physical activity to moderate levels, not from moderate to high levels.*

Thus, the next step might be to test the effectiveness of such messages as, "Just get moving," or, "Walk, don't run!"

SUMMARY

The word "create" means to cause or bring about, to produce, to originate. The creative energy of most practitioners really starts to flow when they reach the point of framing the approach and detailing the tactics that will make up their health promotion program. How do we get that "just right" approach to media advocacy, an innovative policy initiative, or the unique message that reaches people and promotes action heretofore ignored?

While such innovative actions could indeed result from a stroke of creative genius, they are much more likely to be the product of a less dramatic process. This might be the creation of a simpler message, elaborating on a current method, or shifting the emphasis temporarily away from health to a social or economic concern. In this chapter, the underlying message is that the creative process will have a greater chance of leading to effective health promotion tactics if all of the prior steps of the planning process are in alignment.

When things get difficult (and they will) and your program won't work the way you had hoped (and it may not), identify and remember those mistakes long enough to avoid repeating them! Our capacity to learn from false starts is one of the most important and practical steps toward innovation.

ENDNOTES

1. Reid DJ, Killoran AJ, McNeill AD, Chambers JS. Choosing the most effective health promotion option for reducing a nation's smoking prevalence. *Tobacco Control.* 1992;1:185–197. We think that this article offers a very easy-to-follow and practical illustration of how to envision many different methods being applied comprehensively to a single, priority health problem. In the case story, Colonel Gayle's "modified" version of the Reid et al. matrix was easy to create, given the thoughtful detail put into the original.

2. For a clear description of how objectives are critical building blocks for developing effective interventions, we recommend: Puska P, Yuomilehto J, Nissinen A, Vartiainen E. *The North Karelia Project 20-year results and experiences.* Helsinki, Finland: National Public Health Institute and WHO Europe; 1995;44–47.

3. Brownson RC, Koffman DM, Novotny T, Hughes RG, Eriksen MP. Environmental and policy interventions to control tobacco use and prevent cardiovascular disease. *Health Educ Q.* 1995;22(4):478–498.

4. The resources we have used to create this section on health communications are the same resources we turn to in our own planning and research activity: *Making Health Communications Work: A Planner's Guide.* Washington, DC: U.S. Department of Health and Human Services, NIH publication No. 89-1493, 1989; Communication: A Guide for Managers of National Diarrheal Disease Control Programmes. Diarrheal Control Programme, Geneva: World Health Organization, 1987; The CDC Health Communication Book: A Primer on Risk Communication Principles and Practices, Atlanta: Agency for Toxic Substances and Disease Registry, U.S. Department of Health and Human Services, 1994; and Manoff RK, Social Marketing: New Imperative for Public Health, New York: Prager Publishers; 1985.

5. We have chosen to use a "questions" rather than a "steps" format in this context because the latter so often implies a linear, prescribed sequence of actions. We have found that the critical analysis phase of health communication is primarily an interactive process, where insights gained on one issue will trigger revisiting a prior question. To that extent, the priority should not be the order in which questions are asked, just that they are asked in the first place.

6. Some messages may appear to be more compelling, and thus better attended to, than others. For example: "Dangerous Curve, Slow to 15 m.p.h." However, even a message like that could go unattended if it were in a language different from the receiver, or were too small or inadequately lit to be read.

7. Figure 6.2 was taken from *Communication: A Guide for Managers of National Diarrheal Disease Control Programmes.* Geneva, World Health Organization; 1987:30.

8. Maibach E, Parrott RL, eds. *Designing Health Messages.* Thousand Oaks, CA: Sage Publications; 1995.

9. Lefebvre CR, Doner L, Johnston C, Loughrey K, Balch GI, Sutton SM. Use of database marketing and consumer-based health communication in message design. In: Maibach E and Parrott RL, eds. *Designing Health Messages.* Thousand Oaks, CA: Sage Publications; 1995.

10. The "5 a Day" program was initiated in 1988 by the California State Department of Health Service under a grant from the National Cancer Institute

(NCI). The purpose of the program was to promote increases in fruit and vegetable consumption. Based upon the success of the California experience, "5 a Day" became a national campaign in 1991 with the support of the NCI.

11. Kline GF, Pavlik JV. Adolescent health information acquisition from broadcast media. In: Mayer M, ed. *Health Education by Radio and Television.* Munich, Germany: K.G. Saur; 1981:92–117.

12. A full report of the methods and finding of this evaluation can be found in: Kreuter Marshall W, Kreuter Matthew W, Hearn M. *A National Assessment of Reach to Recovery.* Atlanta: American Cancer Society; 1992. The specific reference to the notion of sender credibility is found on page 28 of the report.

13. Green LW, Kreuter MW. *Health Promotion Planning: An Educational and Environmental Approach.* Menlo Park, CA: Mayfield Publishing; 1990:4–5.

14. Chapman S, Lupton D. *The Fight for Public Health: Principles and Practice of Media Advocacy.* London: BMJ Publishing; 1994:135.

15. McKinlay J. A case for refocusing upstream: the political economy of illness. In: Conrad R, Kerns R, eds. *The Sociology of Health and Illness.* New York: St Martin's Press; 1986:484–498.

16. Rose G. *The Strategy of Preventive Medicine.* New York: Oxford University Press; 1992;123–124.

17. For example, see: Wallack L. Mass communication and health promotion: a critical perspective. In: Rice R, Atkin C, eds. *Public Communication Campaigns.* Newbury Park, CA: Sage Publications; 1990; Wallack L, Dorfman L, Jernigan D, Themba M. *Media Advocacy and Public Health: Power for Prevention.* Newbury Park, CA: Sage Publications; 1993; Wallack L, Dorfman L. Television news, hegemony, and health. *Am J Public Health.* 1992;82:125; and Chapman S, Lupton D. *The fight for Public Health: Principles and Practice of Media Advocacy.* London: BMJ Publishing; 1994.

18. Larry Wallack and Lori Dorfman, through the Berkeley Media Studies Group, conduct workshops and training on various aspects of media advocacy. Their work has been featured nationally in many settings, including the Promoting Public Health in an Era of Change training programs sponsored by the User Liaison Program of the Agency for Health Care, and the Kansas Health Foundation's annual Health Leadership Institute.

19. As you consider integrating media advocacy into your mix of health promotion tactics, care not to lose sight of the purpose of media advocacy in public health: to advance or establish healthful policy.

20. For more details on the notion of piggybacking, see: Ryan C. *Prime Time Activism.* Boston: South End Press; 1991; and Wallack L, Dorfman L, Jernigan D, Themba M. *Media Advocacy and Public Health: Power for Prevention.* Newbury Park, CA: Sage Publications; 1993;93.

21. The-wei H, Hai-yen S, Keeler T. Reducing cigarette consumption in California: tobacco taxes versus an anti-smoking media campaign. *Am J Public Health.* 1995;85:1218–1222.

22. Prochaska JO, DiClemente CC. In search of how people change: applications to addictive behaviors. *Am Psychologist.* 1992;47(9):1102–1114; Becker MH (ed.). The health belief model and personal health behavior. *Health Education Monographs.* 1974;2:324–473; and Bandura A. Toward a unifying theory of behavior change. *Psychological Review.* 1977;84(2):191–215.

23. Strecher VJ, Kreuter MW, Den Boer DJ, Korbrin S, Hospers HJ, Skinner CS. The effects of computer-tailored smoking cessation messages in family practice settings. *J Fam Prac.* 1994;39(3):262–270.
24. Rimer BK, Orleans CT, Fleisher L, Cristinzo S, Resch N, Telepchak J, et al. Does tailoring matter? The impact of a tailored guide on ratings and short-term smoking-related outcomes for older smokers. *Health Education Research.* 1994; 9(1):69–84.
25. Campbell MK, DeVellis BM, Strecher VJ, Ammerman AS, DeVellis RF, Sandler RS. The impact of message tailoring on dietary behavior change for disease prevention in primary care settings. *Am J Public Health.* 1994;84(5): 783–787.
26. Skinner CS, Strecher VJ, Hospers H. Physician recommendations for mammography: do tailored messages make a difference? *Am J Public Health.* 1994: 84(1):43–49.
27. Kreuter MW, Vehige E, McGuire AG. Using computer-tailored calendars to promote childhood immunization: a pilot study. *Public Health Reports.* 1996; 111(2).
28. The process of developing tailored messages requires the planner (or team of planners) to have ready access to the following competencies: (1) educational and behavioral theory, (2) data collection (questionnaire design) based on theory, (3) data analysis, (4) creation of multiple messages and testing those messages, and (5) creating the algorithms that will link selected communications and behavioral characteristics with the appropriate message from a library of health messages.
29. It is not our intent to go into detail about the computer programming aspects of tailoring—however, as computer technology in public health continues to expand, practitioners will find it useful to have some conceptual understanding of the process. Step 4 is to develop a database. Once the tailoring assessment has been administered, participants' responses must be recorded in a way that allows them to be easily converted into the appropriate tailored messages. Creating a computer database with at least one data field for each assessment question is the simplest way to do this. Each question in the assessment tool must be assigned a variable name. For example, a question assessing barriers to quitting smoking (such as "What would keep you from quitting smoking?") might be named Q.SMK.BARRIER, shorthand for "question about smoking cessation barriers."

There might be four possible response options to this question: fear of failing, stress, concern about weight gain, and peer pressure; each would be numbered 1, 2, 3, and 4, respectively. So if Jane Doe's record in the database showed a value of 3 in the field named Q.SMK.BARRIER, we would conclude that she said that concern about weight gain might keep her from quitting smoking.

In step 5, the main task is to fit the names of our variables to each tailored message. In the previous step, the barrier for the smoker who was concerned about gaining weight might be called TM.SMK.BAR.WEIGHT, shorthand for "tailored message about smoking cessation barrier weight gain." When all tailored messages have been named, they should be placed together in a single document. This document is the tailored-message library.

Tailoring algorithms are formed by using "if/then" logic statements to join each question variable with its related tailored messages. In our present example, putting these two together gives us an algorithm that might read, "*if* Q.SMK.BARRIER = 3 *then put* TM.SMK.BAR.WEIGHT *in the tailored quit smoking plan.*" In other words, if Jane Doe said concern about weight gain would keep her from quitting, give her the tailored message addressing weight gain as a barrier to cessation.

At its simplest level, tailoring printed materials is nothing more than a complex print-merge function in most word-processing programs. When you send a form letter to 100 different persons using print merge, the letter contains open spaces, or *fields,* for the first name, last name, street address, city, state, and zip. When this letter is merged with a data file containing the names and addresses of the 100 persons, it produces 100 personalized letters. In tailoring, instead of having a small field at the top of the letter allocated to the variable "first name," you might have a field consuming one-third of the page that is allocated to a message about barriers to quitting smoking. When the tailoring algorithms are merged with an individual's responses from the database, the appropriate quit-smoking-barrier message is pulled from the tailored-message library and placed into the participant's feedback.

When all tailoring algorithms have been created, they must be tested extensively. Providing the wrong message to a person (a "tailoring misfire") will not only compromise the credibility of the program, but also could harm the message recipient if inappropriate actions are recommended.

30. Prochaska JO, DiClemente CC, Norcross JC. In search of how people change: applications to addictive behaviors. *Am Psychologist.* 1992;47:1102–1114.
31. Bandura A. *Social Foundations of Thought and Action.* Englewood Cliffs, NJ: Prentice-Hall; 1986.

CHAPTER 7

Steering vs. Rowing

Case Story
JAMESON

Remember the first case story about Linda Thomas? Well, Linda Thomas was not the only one who responded to Fran Martin's remarks about "why we do what we do." Dr. Gordon Jameson—the director of the Tri-county Health Department (TCHD) and Linda Thomas's boss—was also in the audience. Although his given name was Gordon, everyone outside of his professional life called him Jameson—even his mother and father! When he was a young boy he asked his parents why they didn't call him by his given name. They told him that one month after he was born, a very bad man had tried to swindle them out of some property that had been in the family for decades. They explained that it was a nasty encounter that left a lot of bad feelings behind—and the man's name was Gordon. From that point on he was Jameson.

Dr. Martin's remarks had made Jameson recall his magnetic pull to public health two decades before. In addition to being a family practice physician, he had served in the Peace Corps in Ghana. It was his experience in Ghana that convinced him that he could do more good by preventing than by repairing. He had his own handwritten modification to the Hippocratic oath hanging on his office wall: "Do good—do your best to do no harm, and before you do either, ask people if they really want your help in the first place!" He suspected that he shared this "Peace Corps gene" with many of his colleagues.

He wondered, though, if his staff shared these motivations. In fact, he had been troubled throughout Dr. Martin's lecture by a sense that in his own health department, the ideals of public health were not translated into a daily sense of mission and accomplishment. Indeed, he felt a distinct lack of enthusiasm about leaving the glow of her inspiring remarks and returning to the daily grind of the Tri-county Health Department: insufficient resources, staff grievances, media scrutiny, and all the other difficulties that seemed to take up more and more of each day.

Jameson waited patiently as Dr. Martin fielded the usual flurry of inquiries that follow a provocative and stimulating presentation. As a reward for being the last person in line, Jameson suddenly found that he had her

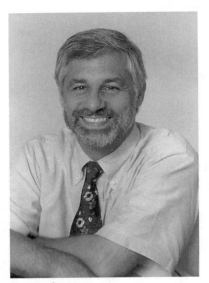

Dr. Gordon Jameson

undivided attention. He introduced himself and told Dr. Martin how much he had appreciated her words, and how he wished more of his staff could have attended the lecture. As their conversation continued, he found himself wondering out loud about whether his staff shared his own views of public health, and whether they, too, felt overwhelmed by the daily struggles their work entailed.

Dr. Martin reassured him that his concerns were far from unique. However, she was not going to let him off the hook that easily. "What are you planning to do about it?" she demanded. Jameson was somewhat taken aback. He had expected to do some more leisurely thinking (and perhaps commiserating!) before taking any action. Besides, he had arranged a management retreat for the staff a few months ago. Somewhat sheepishly, he offered this to Dr. Martin as evidence of his efforts. "A retreat!" she said, in mock horror. "Well," stammered Jameson, trying hard to recover, knowing full well that the retreat had fallen short of his expectations, "Well—I'm open to suggestions!" In the back of his mind, an appealing vision was taking shape—a vision of Dr. Martin swooping into the Tri-county Health Department and motivating the troops.

But swooping was not on Dr. Martin's agenda. "You and your staff are going to have to work on this yourselves," she said, somewhat sternly. "And not during a retreat!" Correctly interpreting the misgivings in his expression, she relented. "I do know some people who could help you get started, though, if you'd like." Dr. Martin jotted down three names on the back of her business card. She circled the middle name and said, "All three of these people are first rate, but this one would be my first choice. He's very insightful, and he's been in the trenches. Best of all, he lives in Atlanta, only 100 miles from your health department—and he *loves* to drive!" Relieved at having a concrete task ahead of him, Jameson thanked Dr. Martin for her remarks and suggestions and agreed to call one of the consultants.

On the first try, Jameson made telephone contact with Bob Del Rey, the man in the middle of Fran Martin's list. Surely, he thought, this was a good sign! When Bob picked up the phone, Jameson was instantly reminded of his own teenage years when he heard—could it be?—ZZ Top blaring in the background. Bob sounded a little out of breath. "Just a minute!" he said, a little louder than necessary. "I'll turn that down!"

When Bob returned to the phone, Jameson explained who he was and how he had ended up calling. They chatted for a few moments about how terrific Fran Martin was, and then Bob asked what Jameson had in mind. Jameson briefly described the size and scope of the health department, and outlined his managerial concerns. Bob asked Jameson to send him some details about the health department's organization, any recent planning documents, and a brief recap of his main concerns. In exchange, Jameson asked Bob to send his résumé. At the end of the conversation, they were on a first-name basis—or, in Jameson's case, close enough!

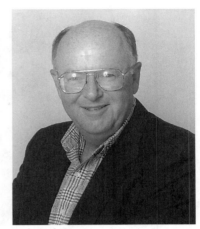

Bob Del Rey

The two men agreed to talk on the phone again after Bob had a chance to review the materials; then Bob would spend two days at the TCHD. Bob proposed to have an initial morning meeting with Jameson alone; then, in the afternoon and on the following day, he would have one-on-one sessions with the supervisors of each major department and a sample of staff throughout the organization. Jameson agreed to make those arrangements.

Meanwhile, Jameson—not doubting Fran Martin's judgment, but intrigued—did some checking on his own. He had a few sources at the CDC, several of whom knew quite a bit about Bob Del Rey. Fortunately, what they had to say was right in line with Dr. Martin's assessment and the information in Bob's résumé.

A graduate of a small liberal-arts college in Iowa, Bob had started out with a commitment to become a dentist, but once his friends asked if he really wanted to spend a lifetime groping around in other people's open mouths, he turned his interest to a more mundane field: biology. Bob graduated on time in 1964 and immediately joined the U.S. Public Health Service, motivated in part by a strong interest in avoiding the war in Vietnam. His first job, as a VD investigator tracking down syphilis cases in New York City, made Bob question his decision to abandon dentistry.

At the time, he had no idea that he would retire 30 years later as one of the most effective managers ever to serve the CDC. Over his three decades of service, Bob accumulated numerous awards and plaques acknowledging his contributions and achievements, none of which ever made it out of the boxes they came in. The only award he displayed was his first-place team trophy for bowling in 1981.

Jameson looked out of his office window just as a red Porsche pulled into the parking lot—right on time for the meeting they had discussed earlier. The consulting business must be a lucrative one for Bob Del Rey,

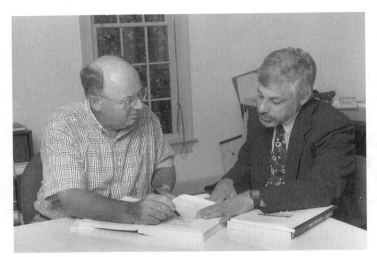

Bob Del Rey and Dr. Gordon Jameson

Jameson thought, although certainly the rates he had quoted seemed very reasonable. Watching curiously and intently, he was surprised to see a man step out of the car, dressed very comfortably in a short-sleeved shirt, loose-fitting khakis, and decidedly nondesigner tennis shoes. He pulled a battered briefcase from the back seat and strode purposefully into the building. Sure enough, the same figure was soon knocking on Jameson's open door.

After he had greeted Jameson with an introductory "Nice to meet you, Gordon," Bob was treated to the story about the swindler. Bob chuckled, "That's a new one!"

After they had seated themselves, Bob hauled a yellow note pad out of his briefcase and readied himself to take a few notes. "I noted in the material you sent," Bob said, "that you had a retreat about six months ago with program managers and came up with vision statements and mission statements for their various programs. Did you also undertake any exercises that resulted in the identification of health priorities in your service area?"

"Actually, yes," Jameson replied. "We asked the directors of four programs—maternal and child health, communicable diseases, nursing, and adult health—to give us annual summaries of the encounters they had by disease or reported health problem. And those matched up pretty well with health objectives outlined in the our state's Healthy People: Health Objectives document."

"Let me ask you a resource question," Bob continued. "In terms of your total TCHD budget, what portions come from local revenues versus state and federal monies?"

Jameson thought for a second and said, "I don't have the exact numbers off the top of my head, but I can give you a pretty accurate estimate. Approximately 40 percent comes from county and municipal revenues. A little over 35 percent comes from state and federal grants and contracts, most of which comes to us through the state health department. We get another 15 percent in fees from services we provide—our well-baby clinics and immunization programs, for example. A small portion falls into the noncategorical area we call *other.*"

"How about the expenditure side?" Bob asked. "Where does the money go?"

"That's easy," Jameson said, recalling frequent testimony to the county commissioners. "Nearly 70 percent goes to salaries, well over 25 percent goes to operating costs, only 1.5 percent goes for capital outlay, and the rest is noncategorical."

Bob nodded. He had known in advance what Jameson's answer would be. Now he changed direction. "OK, of the management challenges you're trying to address, is there any *one* issue or problem that stands out in your mind?"

Jameson's eyes searched the floor for a moment. "I couldn't put my finger on any one issue *per se.* It's just that we always seem to be reacting rather than initiating! Every TCHD employee has a yearly work plan, but I'd bet that over 50 percent of what we actually do is in response to new initiatives or new problems that come up during the year, few of which are in the work plans."

Bob nodded and smiled knowingly. "Other duties as assigned, eh?"

Jameson thought to himself, "I like this guy."

They completed their discussions over lunch. Jameson handed Bob a schedule of meetings with other staff, as Bob had requested. They agreed that, after Bob completed his interviews, he would return to Atlanta, prepare a summary report with recommendations, and have that report back to Jameson within two weeks.

Bob had prepared a series of questions and planned to ask each person the same questions, regardless of his or her department or rank:

- What is the health department's mission?
- What is your division's mission?
- What role do you play in the health department? In your division?
- How long have you been here?
- How are decisions made here?
- What is a typical day like?
- What helps you do your job?
- What hinders you in doing your job?
- What are the main challenges that the health department faces in the next few years?
- How do others, especially those with a stake in health, view the health department and its role?

In addition, as the opportunity presented itself, Bob asked each employee to loosely track how he or she spent every day for a week—an hour-by-hour summary that showed planned and impromptu meetings, new and old crises, paperwork, supervisory commitments, training, and so forth.

Bob Del Rey was easy to talk to. He expressed a sincere interest in people, but was never overbearing. He had the uncanny ability to be frank and kind at the same time. As he listened, he searched for themes and patterns in the responses people gave to his questions. Bob noted that some of those themes echoed the concerns that Jameson had raised during their one-on-one interview. For example, like Jameson, many of the staff felt frustrated by the back-to-back crises that seemed to be hitting them with increasing frequency. Bob also found that some staff were unclear about what the health department's highest priorities should be—even some who had attended the retreat together to craft a mission statement. Indeed, several of those interviewed were unaware that there *was* a new mission statement.

In their comments about the future, staff were concerned about funding cuts and their effects both on their individual jobs and salaries as well as on the health department and its ability to provide needed services. Many felt they were already as lean as they could be, and that the next step would be to have to turn people away or cut back their hours. Staff uniformly acknowledged the sincere dedication Jameson had for his job, and several sympathized with the administrative challenges he faced. As one senior staff member put it, "Who would want his job?"

The staff who saw patients through the department's various clinics also worried that managed-care organizations would underestimate the difficulty of working with populations that the health department had worked with for many years. These staff expressed concerns about whether or not immunizations, HIV counseling and testing, and other needed services would continue at the same levels.

Many staff felt that time and resources were not generally available for attending training or educational sessions, nor did they feel well informed about what other departments were tackling. Some described the frustration they felt when they had trouble explaining what they did to friends or neighbors, especially with the added stigma of working "for the government." When Bob asked staff how others with a stake in health viewed the health department and its role, the responses were vague. Few staff could identify key stakeholders beyond the Board of Health.

Bob was not surprised by the many complaints he heard from staff about the bureaucratic aspects of their jobs—having to fill out forms showing the same data in different ways, writing endless reports for various state and federal agencies, and rarely seeing a return for these efforts. Some suggested that the bureaucracy and funding streams made them inefficient, and that perhaps the health department should be run more like a business. Surely their counterparts in the private sector didn't have to put up with the combination of uncertainty, scrutiny, and disdain that they did!

Bob's conversations with the staff ended on a positive note when they talked about the chains of events—some planned, some completely random—that had led them to this field. In spite of these frustrations, Bob felt that the staff represented a great deal of talent and enthusiasm for public health, and generally respected one another. This was the good news to relay back to the staff and to Jameson.

Bob Del Rey's report back to Jameson was entitled *Opportunities and Challenges for the TCHD*. The introductory section included a brief synthesis of the background information on the TCHD that Jameson had turned over to Bob for review. That was followed by a section called Emerging Issues. Bob had used health status data from the TCHD service area and matched it up with similar indicators for the state of Georgia and for the southeastern region of the United States to make some projections of the health issues most likely to emerge in the TCHD's service area.

The remainder of the report was divided into four components, each of which had been shaped by the information and themes Bob derived from the interviews:

- Essential Services
- Strategic Planning
- Benchmarking
- Private- and Public-Sector Enterprises

For each component, Bob defined the category, explained how staff comments directly or indirectly gave rise to that category, and offered recommendations for action.

In his cover letter to Jameson, Bob included a quote by Max dePree: "The first responsibility of a leader is defining reality."[1]

Bob went on to write:

> In every management situation I can recall over the past 30 years, no single attribute was more critical to building organizational confidence than when the manager or leader was forthcoming with accurate and insightful information about the realities facing the organization. Doubt and mistrust are less likely when leaders seek out and reveal the honest realities of their circumstances, warts included!

Case Analysis

The management "how-to" shelves at bookstores and libraries continue to expand with books on every imaginable managerial challenge. Each book, in turn, adds to the jargon of management. Terms such as Japanese *total quality management* (TQM) and *quality circles* (QCs), *learning organizations, reengineering*, and many others have seeped into our everyday language. Unfortunately, no book—including this one—is going to create good management overnight. Instead, our goal in this section is to examine several basic tenets of good management practice, and ask practitioners to "walk a mile" in the shoes of the supervisor or manager; we have found that practitioners who understand the managerial perspective are more likely than those without such understanding to inform and, in some cases, influence the decisions of their managers and leaders.

We believe that sound management practice is often overlooked, particularly in crisis-driven environments like the TCHD. This occurs for a number of reasons. First, people often assume that managerial skill is a "freebie" that the organization gets with any talented, accomplished person. Unfortunately, skill in one area does not always translate into the managerial realm.

Moreover, training and guidance for managerial functions are often nonexistent or perfunctory—such as a one-day workshop on how to supervise employees or work with a difficult colleague. Another set of assumptions represents the opposite problem—a sort of fatalism about individual styles and personalities and their intractable nature. The fact is that "control freaks" and freewheeling artistic types can all be equally good managers, but they may arrive at that point differently.

The management information presented here is divided into two main categories: organizational and individual. An organization is a collection of individuals who must work together to accomplish common goals. The organization and its leadership have some specific elements to contribute to the organization's success, but so do the individuals who make up the organization. We believe that good management is a collective responsibility of every member of the organization. In this case, for instance, both Linda Thomas and Dr. Jameson have specific contributions to make to the successful management of the TCHD. In other words, even if you are not a manager per se, the management skills outlined here should be useful to you.

MANAGEMENT AND ORGANIZATIONS

Dr. Jameson had already told Bob Del Rey about some of the steps he had taken to define organizational goals. These included the retreat with the department managers, the match between client encounters and published national and state health objectives, and the attempt to create a new mission statement. Unfortunately, Bob's interviews with staff revealed that these efforts had not built consensus throughout the organization. Recall that some people were unaware of the new mission statement, and others disagreed about what the organization's priorities were.

In this section, we will review the following tools and concepts, which were the framework for Bob Del Rey's report:

- essential services of public health
- strategic planning
- benchmarking
- private- and public-sector enterprises

Essential Services

One tool that Dr. Jameson and his staff have not yet used to address these types of discrepancies is the *essential-services* language that we reviewed in Chapter 1. Like the core functions that preceded them, the essential services provide a framework and vocabulary for discussing public health activities. Most organizations will not undertake the entire spectrum of essential services. For example, state and local health departments have different emphases on surveillance (typically heavier at the state level) and personal care services (typically more prevalent at the local level). Community-based organizations, foundations, advocacy groups, hospitals, and others active in public health may each focus on a specific service. In any case, essential-services language offers a way to describe where an organization currently stands and where it might shift in response to its own momentum or the effects of outside forces.

At the TCHD, the essential services could serve as a starting point for discussions about what the TCHD is currently doing, and how this might change in the future. For example, if (as some staff mentioned) managed-care organizations take over some of the services that are currently provided by staff at the TCHD, what will their roles be? The possibilities include collaboration with managed-care organizations (for example, providing outreach services), providing training to staff who are new to population-based services, or even shifting to other services.

Strategic Planning

Anticipating and preparing for the future is an important leadership function for Dr. Jameson and his staff. The process of managing the constant change that affects almost any organization is captured by the *strategic planning* process.[2] *Strategic planning* is a term that is often misused to refer to a specific document—such as the strategic plan that Dr. Jameson sent to Bob Del Rey. A strategic plan *document* is one product of a strategic planning process, but it is by no means the only product, nor is it even the most important one. Many organizations struggle through the long meetings and semantic revisions that lead to a strategic plan, and then breathe a sigh of relief because they believe that they are finished. In fact, the document is a fuzzy snapshot of the organization at a certain point in time, and one that can and should be updated regularly in order to refine the picture and ensure that it remains accurate. Think of the strategic plan itself as a recording or imprint of a dynamic process—something that participants can refer to over time to refresh their memories, check their assumptions, and measure their progress.

Strategic planning can be undertaken in various ways, at various levels of detail. In fact, it may not even be called strategic planning. Regardless of the name it goes by, the strategic planning process tries to answer three key questions: (1) Where are we now? (2) Where do we want to be? and (3) How do we get there? Each of these can have numerous dimensions, such as funding levels, staff skill sets, new products or programs, customer service, collaborative relationships, and so on. These will depend, of course, on the contours of each organization and its subunits. For example, at TCHD, it might be useful for each department to examine these questions, and then to come together as a group to see where there is overlap and/or divergence. See Table 7.1 for common categories addressed through a strategic planning process.

Where Are We Now?

This is the baseline measure of where an organization stands. It typically includes an environmental scan—a sort of lay of the land, internally and externally. An internal assessment takes a clear, unflinching look at the organization's strengths and weaknesses. An external assessment looks at opportunities and threats—which may sometimes be two sides of the same coin. For example, many public health practitioners view the advent of managed-care organizations as both an opportunity and a threat.

Another tool to help determine where an organization stands is sometimes referred to as a *stakeholder analysis*. Who are the key stakeholders for your organization? What do they think of your performance? What criteria do they use to judge your performance?

Where Do We Want To Be?

Future goals should incorporate both short- and long-term time frames—for example, one year as well as four to five years and even a decade into the future. A useful exercise in discussing this question is to have staff think about the future without real-world constraints. Remember Dr. Jameson's "Peace Corps gene"; even goals that sound hopelessly naïve or unrealistic may trigger a useful or just plain inspiring discussion. Perhaps some of those real-world barriers to accomplishing lofty goals are not as imposing or immovable as they seemed. Many good ideas and programs got their start with the words, "If only we could . . ."

How Do We Get There?

Unlike the second question, this one does need to be firmly rooted in reality. What resources are required—money, people, skills, training? What alternative routes are there, if some or all of these are unavailable or are not

TABLE 7.1 Ten Strategic Planning Steps

Step 1: Initiate and Agree on a Strategic Planning Process

- Identify key decision makers
- Determine who should be involved (people, units, agencies)

Step 2: Clarify Organizational Mandates

- List mandates ("musts") and sources (charters, policies, rules)
- Determine implications of mandates for current operations
- Determine whether mandates should be changed

Step 3a: Identify and Understand Stakeholders

- Identify internal and external stakeholders
- Determine criteria they use to judge performance
- Determine how they would rate the agency's performance

Step 3b: Develop/Refine Mission Statement and Values

- Clarify purpose of organization; why you do what you do
- Response to key stakeholders
- Philosophy/core values
- Distinct/unique contributions
- Current values; additional values to guide conduct in the future

Step 4: Assess the Environment

- List *internal* strengths and weaknesses
- List *external* opportunities and threats
- Identify options for building on strengths and opportunities, and minimizing weaknesses and threats

Step 5: Identify/Frame Strategic Issues

- Identify challenges to the organization that require immediate action, action in the near future, or monitoring
- Identify consequences of not addressing each issue

Step 6: Formulate Strategies to Manage Issues

- Determine strategies, barriers, and specific actions to address strategic issues
- Develop a first-draft strategic plan listing specific strategies and actions

Step 7: Review and Adopt the Strategic Plan

- Include key internal and external stakeholders

Step 8: Establish an Effective Organizational Vision for the Future

- Describe the "vision of success" for the organization, based on the mission statement, values, and strategies

Step 9: Develop an Effective Implementation Process

- List existing programs and services
- Set priorities
- Determine actions, results, milestones
- Decide who is responsible
- Assign dates/resources

Step 10: Reassess the Strategic Planning Process

- Identify strengths and weaknesses of existing strategies
- Suggest modifications
- Decide which should be maintained, revised, or terminated

available in the quantities needed? What kinds of new or reinforced collaboration may be required? And the most important questions: Who will be responsible for it, and by when? This is the most important part of the written document. It is acceptable to miss these deadlines, but it is also acceptable to expect an explanation—and a modification for the next round of goals and timelines. If timelines and responsibilities are agreed upon and nothing else ever happens, your next planning effort will have to surmount a lot of skepticism—as well it should.

Benchmarking

You have probably noticed that answers to each of these questions depend on some type of objective measures of what the current situation is, and how it changes over time. The national Healthy People objectives for the nation are one such measure. As Dr. Jameson pointed out, these have been adapted by many states for their own specific circumstances. The Oregon benchmarks process described in Chapter 2 is an excellent example of how measurable goals are used to drive activities not only in public health but throughout state government. If Bob Del Rey had asked TCHD counterparts in Oregon about their organization's goals, chances are they would have been able to provide a succinct list for each department.

Private- and Public-Sector Enterprises

The TCHD staff members interviewed by Bob Del Rey talked about two common aspects of working for a government agency: the frustration of internal bureaucratic procedures and the stigma that outsiders attach to "government work."

More and more politicians find it fashionable to be critical of public agencies and public service; they paint pictures of Kafkaesque bureaucratic nightmares featuring anecdotes of wasteful government spending and intrusive regulations. Without engaging in the debate over how much or how little government is enough, suffice it to say that in the realm of public health, government agencies at all levels have quietly and successfully assumed responsibility for a wide variety of health issues that affect us as individuals and as communities.

Public health is a public good—one that we benefit from simultaneously as individuals and as communities. It is certainly in your individual interest that the man standing next to you in line at the bus stop not suffer from tuberculosis. It happens to also be in the interests of the other people in the same line, and everyone else who may come into casual contact with him throughout the day. However, there is no profit incentive to induce a private organization to worry about this. Public health does worry about it, and tries to do something about it.

As David Osborne and Ted Gaebler point out in their book, *Reinventing Government,* the differences between government and business enterprises "add up to one conclusion: Government cannot be run like a business."[3] One of the differences they cite is the slower pace of government, since decisions must be made more openly and with far more outside scrutiny than in business. Another important distinction is that government cannot choose its customers; by definition, government agencies must serve everyone equally. (In public health, this has historically meant those customers least able to afford and acquire health care services elsewhere—those who are often most resource-intensive.) Flexibility in hiring (and firing) staff is restricted in public agencies. Finally, as a Ford Foundation official notes in Osborne and Gaebler's book, "In government, all of the incentive is in the direction of not making mistakes. You can have 99 successes and nobody notices, and one mistake and you're dead."

This is not to say that government enterprises can't be improved—certainly they can. In fact, that is the main point of Osborne and Gaebler's book. But no matter how much government enterprises can adapt and benefit from private-sector management techniques and entrepreneurial spirit, the fact remains that there are fundamental differences between the two.

What does all this have to do with management? It has to do with working with what you have. At the TCHD, some of the problems that staff identified could certainly be improved. These include trying to streamline data collection and reporting (perhaps making better use of automation, if the forms and duplication are not in the TCHD's control).

Another topic that staff identified was the view that outsiders have of their work. In Chapter 4, the point was made that a sizable portion of the public is unaware of what public health really does. Certainly a key management task is to keep stockholders cognizant of what you are doing, so that the recipients of the information see how they and the community benefit. Identifying and understanding stockholders—both internal and external—is a critical step in the strategic planning process outlined in Table 7.1. In addition to stakeholder analysis, addressing this could involve helping staff communicate with the media and with community members about the services they provide.

Staff should pursue these and other improvements with commitment and energy. However, they must also recognize the constraints of their environment. Indeed, the TCHD cannot be run like a business. This means that some efficiencies and resources are lost. But it also has a positive aspect emanating from the organization's mission and contributions to the public's health.

MANAGEMENT AND INDIVIDUALS

The human element of the workplace can be its most rewarding as well as its most frustrating feature. Our work lives would certainly be dull if we worked alongside professionals who had no idiosyncrasies or variation. On the other hand, some personal and professional characteristics can be annoying or even destructive—both to individual colleagues and to the delicate "social fabric" of teams.

What are individuals' obligations to a well-managed organization? We believe these fall into several categories, which are discussed in the following sections:

- information flow
- the supervisory relationship
- professional development
- professional identity

Information Flow

The flow of information is radically transforming every aspect of daily life, including the workplace. Computers, with their vast storage and processing capabilities, and now the information superhighway have made instant access to information the norm for many.

What does this mean for how organizations are managed? One implication is a pressure (and capability) to decentralize decision making, since there is not enough time to pass information up and down a hierarchy. But it also means that individuals are inundated and often overwhelmed with information. The task before them is to wade through piles of papers (and now hundreds of Web sites) to decide which of these many pieces of information are actually relevant.

The flow of information within an organization is a clear juncture of organizational and individual responsibilities. In the TCHD example, Dr. Jameson and his senior staff need to do a better job of communicating their own sense of priorities and mission to "the troops." But the troops also have a role to play. If you find yourself in the position that Linda Thomas was in, without much strategic direction for your ideas and enthusiasm, you now have the tools to request more information from others in the organization. In other words, you should ask yourself *and others*: Why are we doing this? How will it help us accomplish our objectives? Is this a better use of resources than another project? Why or why not?

Another aspect of information flow is almost too trite to mention. In any organization, rumors about individuals and about organizations can develop a life of their own, often to the detriment of individual reputations and organizational effectiveness. At the TCHD, uncertainty about the future creates a ripe climate for this kind of negative speculation. While a certain amount of this is inevitable, much can be avoided by making as much information as possible available to the greatest number of people. Obviously, personnel decisions and other matters must be treated confidentially. However, the results of the strategic planning retreat, the mission statement, even a frank discussion of what the future might hold—all of these can help allay unnecessary fears among staff. Although Bob Del Rey did not feel that morale was anywhere near a crisis stage at TCHD, he did recognize some early warning signs—and he knew the remedy.

The Supervisory Relationship

Solid supervisory skills are the building blocks of good managerial practice, since they govern the one-on-one interactions as well as the teams that make up an organization. Specific supervisory roles vary depending on the organization, but most include the following responsibilities:

- planning and organizing the work that needs to be done
- managing people—hiring, training, informing, supporting, and evaluating them
- achieving objectives—making sure that plans are efficiently implemented, setting performance standards, and adapting to changing conditions.

There is no single path to being a good supervisor; supervisory styles span a wide array of personality types and styles. No matter what the specific responsibilities and individual styles, though, several aspects of good supervision are necessary:

Know your job and your organization. Familiarity with the organization's mission, procedures, and functions is essential to monitoring resources and guiding employees.

Maintain high standards for your own performance. Supervisors need to call upon a range of conceptual, communications, and technical skills. Make sure that your contributions are of the highest caliber.

Lead by example. Model the high standards and professional behavior you expect of your employees, including timeliness, focus, quality control, fairness, and honesty . . . among many others.

Delegate effectively. Peter Drucker, the management "guru," has said that "the purpose of delegation is to enable the supervisor to concentrate on his or her own job, not to delegate it away." Appropriate delegation frees up thinking and planning time, gives other employees an opportunity to learn new skills, demonstrates trust and confidence, and can improve decision making by bringing in new ideas and perspectives. Routine tasks, technical issues, and tasks with potential for skill building are all good candidates for delegation. However, delegation is not always the answer. Do not delegate sensitive personnel matters, those requiring confidentiality, crises, or activities that someone expects you (specifically) to complete.

Professional Development

In order to do their jobs well, staff need to improve their own skills. Some of this can happen through individual initiative, but organizations have an obligation to identify these needs and act on them. Even when limited budgets and scheduling difficulties hinder attendance at conferences and other training events, professional development can still occur. Opportunities include bringing outside trainers in to work with a group from a city or region, using satellite or video capabilities to transfer knowledge (followed by an interactive discussion among participants on site), and holding informal brown-bag lunches to share new information or ideas.

Ideally, professional development is tied to individual performance through the performance review process, during which individual staff members work with their supervisors to identify areas where training would be helpful. A secondary step is to assess training needs across the organization, to see which might be relevant to a group of people or to a particular time in their careers.

Professional Identity

Each of us brings a professional persona to the workplace, composed in part of our personality, our previous work experience, and the influence of a particular discipline or training—among many other factors. Each organization also has expectations of what constitutes professional (and unprofessional) behavior, whether these are articulated or not. In discussing this often implicit aspect of the workplace, Bob Del Rey often mentioned an example from his wife's work as a kindergarten teacher. As a group, Bob's wife and her colleagues got together to decide what it meant to be a professional kindergarten teacher. Their list was not long—in fact, it easily fit on a page. It was a pithy statement of what they valued about their professional identity and what they expected of each other in dealing with peers, students, parents, and school administrators. Again, this is a useful exercise for any group of people working together, since many of these assumptions may not be equally self-evident to everyone.

SUMMARY

Why do we do what we do? This is the question that opened this book, and the one we have returned to in this final chapter. Public health practitioners are fortunate to work in a field that many consider a calling—one that combines compassion for others with elements of activism, innovation, and challenge. However, even the most motivated individuals and the most well-intentioned leaders of organizations can falter when they try to translate their enthusiasm and interests into day-to-day practice.

In this chapter, we have presented some tools for gauging an organization's health, setting priorities, and managing how work gets done. We believe that it is important for everyone in an organization to understand how they contribute to the organization's work. In this sense, solid management is not solely the responsibility of the organization's leaders and senior staff. While managers may do more steering than rowing, it is important for *all* employees to do a little of both—and to know when each is appropriate.

We hope that each of the chapters in this book has helped you formulate your own answers to Fran Martin's probing question, and that you will apply this insight as you put *Ideas that Work* to work in your community.

Good luck!

ENDNOTES

1. dePree, M. *Leadership is an Art,* Doubleday/Currency, New York. 1989.
2. An excellent strategic planning resource is: Bryson J. *Strategic Planning for Public and Nonprofit Organizations.* San Francisco: Jossey-Bass; 1995. The accompanying workbook, *Creating and Implementing Your Strategic Plan,* provides sample worksheets and exercises for conducting a strategic planning process.
3. Osborne D, Gaebler T. *Reinventing Government: How the Entrepreneurial Spirit is Transforming the Public Sector.* Reading, MA: Addison-Wesley; 1992.

Index